MILADY®
STANDARD COSMETOLOGY

THEORY
WORKBOOK

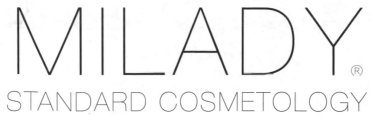

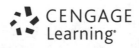

CENGAGE
Learning®

Australia • Brazil • Japan • Korea • Mexico • Singapore • Spain • United Kingdom • United States

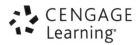

CONTENTS

INTRODUCTION

Congratulations! As a student of cosmetology you now hold in your hands an important tool designed to help you successfully progress through your course of study. You have chosen to embark upon a career in cosmetology, and that can be a life-transforming event. In this journey, you deserve the best possible education, and that can be accomplished by using the best possible educational tools available. The *Milady Standard Cosmetology Theory Workbook* is one of those tools. The *Theory Workbook* has been written to meet the needs, interests, and abilities of students receiving training in cosmetology.

Purpose

The purpose of the *Milady Standard Cosmetology Theory Workbook* is to act as a study tool for you to achieve the objectives of each lesson presented by your instructors. Each chapter is designed to accompany the textbook chapters you will be assigned in the *Milady Standard Cosmetology* textbook. The workbook is comprised of written questions including essay, fill-in-the-blank, true/false, multiple choice, and matching. Each chapter includes an extra activity that may require additional research or completion of a subject-related project to help reinforce your understanding of the textbook.

HOW TO USE THIS WORKBOOK

This workbook should be used with the *Milady Standard Cosmetology* textbook and the *Milady Standard Cosmetology Practical Workbook*. This workbook directly follows the theoretical information found in your textbook. Pages to be read and studied prior to filling out the workbook exercises are listed at the beginning of each chapter. Additional practical information and exercises can be found in the *Milady Standard Cosmetology Practical Workbook*.

The best practice is to close your textbook and see how much you have retained after reading the chapter and taking part in the classroom lessons presented by your instructor. Answer each question in this workbook with a pencil after consulting your textbook for the correct information. The questions can be corrected and/or rated during class or individually. Consult with your instructor to ensure that you are using this workbook in the manner intended and to determine how credit will be awarded for your completion of the exercises contained herein.

Date: _____

Rating: _____

Text Pages: 4–19

1. What is the term used to encompass a broad range of specialty areas, including hairstyling, nail technology, and esthetics? _____

   _____

2. Define cosmetology. _____

   _____

3. What Greek word is the term *cosmetology* derived from? _____

   What does this term mean? _____

why study COSMETOLOGY HISTORY & CAREER OPPORTUNITIES?

4. In your own words, describe why you think it is important for you to learn about old and ancient techniques that were once used in cosmetology.

   _____

   _____

   _____

   _____

   _____

   _____

5. Cosmetologists who know something about the history of their profession are better able to _____ and understand upcoming trends.

Understand the History of Cosmetology

6. What natural products did ancient people use for coloring matter and tattooing?

   _____

7. African civilization had a variety of hairstyles and they were used as a symbol of tribal traditions and conveyed a message of age, marital status, power, and

   _____.

8. What did many African tribes color their hair with? _____

9. What was the first civilized culture to cultivate beauty into an extravagant fashion?
   _____ For what purposes did they use cosmetics?

   _____

   _____

10. As early as 2630 BC, Egyptians used all of the following to create makeup for their eyes, lips, and skin except _____ .

    _____ a) bones   _____ c) insects

    _____ b) berries   _____ d) minerals

11. _____ was an ancient queen who used custom-blended essential oils as signature scents.

12. Which Egyptian queen had a personal cosmetics factory?

    _____

13. In both ancient Egypt and Rome, military commanders stained their nails and lips in matching colors before important battles.

    _____ True   _____ False

14. What did Chinese aristocrats rub onto their nails to color them crimson or ebony?

    _____

15. During the Chou Dynasty, what might have happened to commoners caught wearing a royal nail color?

    _____

16. Throughout the Chou Dynasty, _____ were the royal colors.

    _____ a) black and red   _____ c) gold and silver

    _____ b) purple and blue   _____ d) silver and bronze

17. In 500 BC, during the Golden Age of _____, hairstyling became a highly developed art.

18. Greek women applied preparations of _____ onto their faces, _____ around their eyes, and _____ on their cheeks and lips.

19. How did the Greeks create the brilliant red pigment named vermillion?

_____

20. In Rome, women used hair color to indicate their class in society. Match the correct shade with its corresponding class:

_____ 1) Noblewomen   _____ a) Black

_____ 2) Middle-class women   _____ b) Red

_____ 3) Poor women   _____ c) Blond

21. Facials made of milk and bread, fine wine, corn with flour and milk, or flour and fresh butter, were popular with the:

_____ a) Greeks   _____ c) Romans

_____ b) Chinese   _____ d) Egyptians

22. During the Middle Ages, what part of the face did women not wear colored makeup?

_____ a) Lips   _____ b) Cheeks   _____ c) Eyes

23. Which of the following techniques was refined by a physician during the Middle Ages?

_____ a) Croquignole wrapping technique   _____ c) Henna-based hair dyes

_____ b) Steam distillation   _____ d) Cold waving

24. Beauty culture in the Middle Ages is evidenced by sculptures, _____, and other artifacts from this period.

25. What was discouraged during the Renaissance? _____

_____

26. During the Renaissance, women shaved their eyebrows and hairlines to appear _____.

27. During the Victorian Age, what did women use to preserve the health and beauty of the skin? _____ What were they made from?

_____

28. What did Victorian women do to induce natural color rather than use cosmetics?

_____

29. List two major developments that occurred in the early twentieth century that changed Americans' ideas about beauty.

1) _____

2) _____

30. Why was Max Factor's makeup popular with movie stars?

_____

31. _____ invented a heavily wired machine that supplied electrical current to metal rods around which hair strands were wrapped.

32. Which of the following methods was most appropriate for use on long hair during the waving process?

_____ Croquignole wrapping   _____ Spiral wrapping

33. Check which of the following achievements were attained by Sarah Breedlove?

_____ a) Organizing one of the first national meetings for businesswomen in the United States

_____ b) Inventing the curling iron

_____ c) Pioneering the modern African American hair care and cosmetics industry

_____ d) Devising sophisticated sales and marketing strategies for her hair care products

_____ e) Inventing ammonia-free haircolor

34. Who invented the curling iron? _____

35. _____ advertisements were initially considered _____ by many women's magazines in the early 1920s.

36. Charles Revson borrowed formulas from what industry to develop his nail polish?

_____

37. Name two movie stars who helped make nail polish popular in the 1930s.

_____

38. The _____ was introduced in 1932 by the company Clairol.

39. Today's alkaline perms are modern versions of what method of permanent waving developed in 1941? _____

40. A term used today that refers to the variety of permanent waving and straightening services available for various hair types and conditions is called _____ services.

41. This stylist shook the beauty world in the 1960s with his geometric cuts.

_____

42. During the 1970s there was a new era in highlighting when French hairdressers introduced the art of hair weaving using _____.

43. Which of the following best describes the use of beauty products during the 1980s?

_____ a) Barely there

_____ b) Heavy on the eye shadow and blush

_____ c) Gentle haircolors in many shades

_____ d) Dark lipstick colors

44. The twenty-first century is currently considered the age of _____ in the beauty industry.

45. Name the event held for the first time in 1989 with only five categories for awards.

_____

46. Since the late 1980s, the salon industry has evolved to include _____, a term first coined by Noel DeCaprio.

Learn the Importance of Continuing Education

47. List four ways to take advantage of continuing education.

1) _____

2) _____

3) _____

4) _____

Discover the Career Paths for Cosmetologists

48. In addition to attending school, a cosmetologist must be _____ to work as a professional.

49. List at least eight different areas you may specialize in within the professional industry. The first one is provided to help you get started.

    1) Haircolor specialist.

    2) _____

    3) _____

    4) _____

    5) _____

    6) _____

    7) _____

    8) _____

    9) _____

    10) _____

    11) _____

50. It is a good idea for a haircutting specialist to _____ with other reputable _____ as a way of perfecting his or her technique.

51. The career possibilities can be endless for a hard-working professional cosmetologist who continues their education and approaches his or her career with a strong sense of _____.

52. The salon industry relies heavily on its relationships with _____ in order to stay abreast of what is occurring in the marketplace.

53. Having a strong public speaking ability is important for this beauty professional.

    _____

54. If you choose a career as a film, theatrical, or editorial stylist, you may need to join a(n) _____.

55. Explain which of the specialized areas you are most interested in and why.

    _____

    _____

    _____

    _____

56. Describe the skills required of a salon manager.

_____

_____

_____

_____

_____

57. The salon business typically _____ recessions better than other industries.

58. List ways you can make each day in school have a positive impact on your future.

_____

_____

_____

_____

59. Your license will unlock countless doors, but what two things will determine how successful you become? _____

60. **ACTIVITY:** After thoroughly reviewing this chapter, conduct an Internet research on the history of cosmetology. Write a brief report, about three or four paragraphs in length, explaining which era and/or which individual you believe has had the greatest influence on the field of cosmetology as we know it today.

_____

_____

_____

_____

_____

_____

_____

_____

_____

2 LIFE SKILLS

Date: _____

Rating: _____

Text Pages: 20–35

1. The salon is a creative workplace where you will exercise your _____, and it is a highly social environment that influences workers to develop exceptional communication, decision-making, image-building, customer service, _____, goal-setting, and time management skills.

why study LIFE SKILLS?

2. Practicing good life skills will lead to a more _____ and _____ beauty career.

3. Describe in your own words why you think having good life skills will help build your self-esteem.

_____

_____

_____

_____

Life Skills in Action

4. Below is a list of different life skills. Put a check mark next to the skills you feel you are well on your way to mastering, and put a circle next to the ones you need to improve.

_____

_____

_____

_____

_____ Being caring and helpful to others

_____ Making good friends

_____ Feeling good about yourself

_____ Having a sense of humor to bring you through difficult situations

_____ Maintaining a cooperative attitude

_____ Approaching work with a strong sense of responsibility

_____ Being consistent with your work

_____ Successfully adapting to different situations

_____ Sticking to a goal and seeing a job through to completion

_____ Mastering techniques that will help you become more organized

_____ Developing sound decision-making skills

Interpret the Psychology of Success

5. The process of _____, or fulfilling your full potential, requires lifelong commitment. Stay the course and pursue your success by fueling your

   _____.

6. List the 10 action steps to create a solid foundation for achieving your goals.

   1) _____

   2) _____

   3) _____

   4) _____

   5) _____

   6) _____

   7) _____

   8) _____

   9) _____

   10) _____

7. How is self-esteem related to success? _____

   _____

8. What will help you turn your vision into realities? _____

_____

9. How can you maintain a positive self-image? _____

_____

10. *Success* has been defined in many ways over the years. How do you define success?

_____

_____

_____

_____

11. What is one method for developing success? _____

_____

12. What is a counterproductive activity in the salon? _____

_____

13. Circle each correct answer. Successful stylists (do / do not) take care of themselves; they (do / do not) not get the proper amount of sleep. They (do / do not) create balance by spending time with family and friends, having hobbies, and enjoying recreational activities.

14. List three ways to show respect for others.

1) _____

2) _____

3) _____

15. Unscramble each term and then match it with its definition.

naotiostcrinpra   mfepnictsioer   eagm apln

_____   To put off until tomorrow what you can do today

_____   The unhealthy compulsion to do things perfectly

_____   The conscious act of planning your life, instead of just letting things happen

16. To achieve success, you need more than an _____ because you are the one in charge of managing your own life and learning.

17. In order to manage your own life and learning successfully, you must use
_____.

18. Explain what is meant by creativity.

_____

_____

_____

19. Name four guidelines to follow to enhance your creativity.

1) _____

2) _____

3) _____

4) _____

20. Why is it important to be positive? _____

_____

21. What does "improve your vocabulary" mean? _____

_____ Give some examples. _____

_____

22. What is a mission statement?

_____

_____

_____

_____

23. Write a personal mission statement that communicates who you are and what you want in life.

_____

_____

_____

_____

Set Goals

24. What is the purpose of setting goals?

_____

_____

25. Why is it important to map out your goals?

_____

_____

26. When setting goals, categorize them based on the amount of _____ it takes to accomplish them.

27. Describe the difference between short-term goals and long-term goals.

_____

_____

28. List five short-term goals and five long-term goals and the actions required to achieve them.

	Short-Term Goals	Action
1		
2		
3		
4		
5		

	Long-Term Goals	Action
1		
2		
3		
4		
5		

29. When larger _____ are divided into short-term goals, each step leads to the accomplishment of a larger goal.

30. Remember to set _____ goals, to create a plan of action, and to _____ the plan often.

31. An average person spends _____ checking e-mail, looking at websites, or watching videos each day.

_____ a) one hour   _____ c) four hours

_____ b) three hours   _____ d) six hours

Demonstrate Time Management

32. All people have a(n) _____ that helps them manage their time efficiently if they pay attention to it.

33. Read through the time management techniques listed below. For each, check whether you feel the technique is a strength or an area you need to develop or improve.

_____

_____

_____

_____

Time-Management Techniques	Strength	Development Opportunity
Prioritizing tasks		
Designing my own time management system		
Not taking on more than I can handle		
Learning problem-solving techniques		
Giving myself down time		
Having a notepad, organizer, tablet, or other digital application accessible at all times		
Making schedules for my regular commitments		
Knowing personal energy levels throughout the day		
Rewarding myself for good work		
Using to-do lists to prioritize tasks and activities		
Including time for physical activity		
Scheduling at least one block of free time each day		
Making effective time management a habit		

Employ Successful Learning Tools

34. List key learning tools that should be employed while in school.

    a) _____

    b) _____

    c) _____

    d) _____

    e) _____

    f) _____

    g) _____

    h) _____

35. Discuss why it is important for you to continue to seek educational opportunities after you have completed school.

    _____

    _____

    _____

36. If you find studying overwhelming what can you do?

    _____

37. What can you do if you find your mind wanders in class?

    _____

    _____

38. List the habits you can develop to improve your study skills.

    Where

    _____

    _____

    _____

    When

    _____

    _____

_____

_____

How

_____

_____

_____

Practice Ethical Standards

39. The moral principles by which we live and work are _____.

40. List the five professional behaviors that will show you are an ethical person.

    1) _____

    2) _____

    3) _____

    4) _____

    _____

    5) _____

41 Describe how to maintain your integrity.

    _____

42. Nancy had a fight with her daughter before going to work at the salon;
    she recounts the entire fight with her first client of the morning.
    What is Nancy demonstrating?

    _____ a) Her honesty and directness with everyone because she speaks her mind

    _____ b) Her ability to provide self-care by venting her feelings

    _____ c) Her lack of discretion by sharing a personal issue with a client

43. Your responsibility to behave ethically extends to your _____ with
    customers and coworkers.

44. To be helpful to others, it is essential to take _____.

45. It would be _____ not to recommend certain products or services that
    would be beneficial to a client.

Develop a Positive Personality and Attitude

46. List the characteristics of a healthy, positive attitude.

_____

_____

47. What does *diplomacy* mean?

_____

48. When is assertiveness no longer a positive quality?

_____

49. Learning how to handle a confrontation and how to share your feelings in a professional manner are important indicators of _____.

50. Our behavior and direction are guided by our _____.

51. Taking the time to really listen to others as well as being open-minded and willing to work with all personality types greatly improve an individual's

_____.

52. In both your business and personal life, a pleasing attitude gains more associates, clients, and friends. Think about what having a "pleasing attitude" means to you personally, and describe some ways you can work toward improving your attitude.

_____

_____

_____

_____

_____

_____

_____

53. (W) **ACTIVITY:** Reflect on the content of this chapter and design a personal time management system that will work effectively for you. Consider your flexibility or lack thereof. Consider your ability to say no to others. Determine if you need to improve your problem-solving techniques. Think about what you need to do to remain positive, such as daily self-talk. Think about your daily schedule and how to document it. List the types of rewards you would like to give yourself when you achieve a success. Do not forget to consider your priorities. List the key elements of your personal time management system below.

_____

_____

_____

_____

_____

_____

_____

_____

_____

_____

_____

CHAPTER 3 YOUR PROFESSIONAL IMAGE

Date: _____

Rating: _____

Text Pages: 36–45

1. List the five components that help create a recipe for success.

   1) _____

   2) _____

   3) _____

   4) _____

   5) _____

why study THE IMPORTANCE OF YOUR PROFESSIONAL IMAGE?

2. List at least four reasons why cosmetologists should study and have a thorough understanding of the importance of their professional image.

   1) _____

   _____

   _____

   2) _____

   _____

   _____

   3) _____

   _____

   _____

   4) _____

   _____

Apply Healthful Habits in Your Daily Routine

3. Where does being well groomed begin? _____

4. Why is practicing good personal hygiene so important in the beauty business?

   _____

   _____

5. It is necessary to do which of the following every day?

   _____ a) Shower or bathe   _____ c) Wear perfume

   _____ b) Shampoo your hair   _____ d) Polish your nails

6. _____ is the daily maintenance of cleanliness by practicing good, healthful habits.

7. Working as a stylist, makeup artist, nail technician, or esthetician means that you will be _____ clients.

   _____ a) in close proximity to   _____ c) referred to others by all

   _____ b) highly regarded by all   _____ d) less than friendly with all

8. One of the best ways to ensure that you always smell fresh and clean is to create a _____ to use at work. List the items that should be included.

   _____

   _____

9. While working in a salon, when is it necessary for you to wash your hands?

   _____ a) Before each service   _____ c) After applying moisturizing lotion

   _____ b) Whenever you feel like it   _____ d) After applying nail polish

10. What should you do if you smoke?

    _____

    _____

Follow Image Building Basics

11. Many salon owners and managers view _____ and _____ as being just as important as technical knowledge and skills.

12. The process of caring for parts of the body and maintaining an overall polished look is known as _____.

13. Personal grooming habits are reflected in how a person dresses and takes care of his or her _____, _____, and _____.

14. Which is an extremely important element of your professional image?

_____ a) Personal relationships   _____ c) Clean and stain free clothes

_____ b) Expensive shears   _____ d) Designer clothes

15. Explain why it is a good idea to invest in an apron or a smock.

_____

_____

16. Everyone has a unique personality that is reflected through clothing, shoes, and accessories. While working, cosmetology professionals must remember to tune that style in to the salon's _____.

17. When shopping for work clothes, _____ how you would look in them while performing services.

18. List the universal wardrobe guidelines below.

a) _____

_____

b) _____

_____

c) _____

_____

d) _____

_____

e) _____

_____

19. Why is it important to complement your wardrobe with an up-to-date hairstyle?

_____

_____

20. A cosmetologist wears sunscreen regularly as part of the ongoing process of maintaining healthy skin.

_____ True   _____ False

21. Why are ill-fitting shoes or high heels not the best choice for a cosmetologist?

_____

_____

22. Makeup should be used to _____ facial features.

23. Beauty industry professionals have the privilege of using their hands to make a living, and rarely neglect their own care.

_____ True _____ False

24. A positive attitude is one of the _____ in developing a professional image.

25. When using social media websites to promote your business, be sure to post helpful content, avoid the use of profane language, do not participate in or entertain arguments online, and never post _____ photographs.

26. Politeness is the hallmark of professionalism, even when under _____ .

Employ Proper Ergonomics to Protect Your Body

27. _____ is an important part of your physical presentation. Why?

_____

_____

_____

_____

28. List the guidelines for achieving and maintaining good posture.

_____

_____

_____

_____

29. Define ergonomics.

_____

_____

_____

_____

30. Give an example of fitting the job to the person in the salon.

_____

_____

_____

_____

31. The best way to avoid problems of the hands, wrists, shoulders, neck, back, feet, and legs is to _____ them from occurring in the first place.

32. Repetitive motions can have a cumulative effective on the muscles and joints of the body.

_____ True   _____ False

33. List the bad habits that should be monitored to avoid repetitive motion problems.

a) _____

_____

b) _____

_____

c) _____

_____

d) _____

_____

e) _____

_____

34. What measures can you take to avoid these problems?

a) _____

_____

b) _____

_____

c) _____

_____

d) _____

_____

e) _____

_____

f) _____

_____

35. How can you counter the negative impact of repetitive motions or long periods spent in one position?

_____

36. You should always put your health and well-being first.

_____ True   _____ False

37. ⬤ **ACTIVITY:** Conduct research regarding how the Occupational Safety and Health Administration (OSHA) governs and monitors ergonomics. You can find this information by going to the OSHA website (www.osha.gov) and in the search box type in "ergonomics." After reviewing the information on the website, answer the following questions:

_____

_____

a) How are musculoskeletal disorders (MSDs) defined?

_____

_____

_____

b) What are some of the causes of MSDs in the workplace?

_____

_____

_____

c) Explain the responsibility of employers to protect workers.

_____

_____

_____

d) Why is training an important element in the ergonomic process?

_____

_____

_____

e) List some examples of MSDs.

_____

_____

_____

4 COMMUNICATING FOR SUCCESS

Date: _____

Rating: _____

Text Pages: 46–65

1 List three things that effective human relations and communication skills will help.

1) _____

2) _____

3) _____

why study COMMUNICATING FOR SUCCESS?

2. List seven reasons why it is important for cosmetologists to study and have a thorough understanding of communicating for success.

1) _____

_____

2) _____

_____

3) _____

_____

4) _____

_____

5) _____

_____

6) _____

_____

7) _____

_____

Practice Communication Skills

3. Most of a stylist's _____ will depend on his or her ability to communicate successfully with a wide range of people.

4. The key to operating effectively in many professions is to understand _____. Why is it especially true for cosmetologists?

_____

5. List five practical steps for effectively communicating in the workplace and explain what each one means to you.

1) _____

_____

_____

_____

_____

_____

_____

_____

_____

2) _____

_____

_____

_____

_____

_____

_____

_____

_____

3) _____

_____

_____

_____

_____

_____

_____

_____

4) _____

_____

_____

_____

_____

_____

_____

_____

5) _____

_____

_____

_____

_____

_____

_____

_____

6. What is one strategy for dealing with an aggressive client?

_____ a) Fight back   _____ c) Agree with him or her

_____ b) Turn the other cheek   _____ d) Refuse to continue the service

7. List the golden rules of communication to build a successful beauty industry career.

a) _____

b) _____

c) _____

d) _____

e) _____

f) _____

8. Define effective communication.

_____

_____

9. Besides communicating with words, how else do people communicate?

_____

10. Communicate professionally by using the _____ and thoroughly explaining the features and benefits of the products and services provided.

11. How should you act the first time you meet a client?

_____ a) Polite, friendly, and aloof

_____ b) Polite, genuinely friendly, and inviting

_____ c) Friendly, inviting, and distant

_____ d) Casual, friendly, and solemn

12. Explain the steps you need to take to earn new clients' trust and loyalty.

a) _____

_____

_____

b) _____

_____

_____

13. Every new client should fill out a client intake form, also called a _____, _____, or health history form.

14. The client's permanent progress record of services received including allergies or sensitivities, results, formulations, and products used during the service or purchased for home use is called the _____.

_____ a) client service ticket   _____ c) service record card

_____ b) client service receipt   _____ d) client progress file

15. Why is the intake form a valuable source of information about a client?

_____

_____

_____

_____

16. In some cosmetology schools, the client intake form may be accompanied by a

_____. What is its purpose?

_____

_____

17. A new client should arrive approximately _____ ahead of his or her appointment to complete the client intake form.

Conducting the Client Consultation

18. What is the purpose of the client consultation?

_____

_____

19. The client consultation is one of the most important parts of any service.

_____ True   _____ False

20. How often should a client consultation be performed?

_____ a) Never   _____ c) Every other visit

_____ b) Every visit   _____ d) Only during the first visit

21. A happy client means _____ for both you and the salon.

22. How can you make the most of the client consultation dialogue?

_____

23. What items should you have on hand for use in the client consultation?

a) _____

b) _____

c) _____

d) _____

24. One key to a successful client consultation is making sure the consultation area is
_____ and uncluttered.

25. The following list is the 10-Step Consultation Method. In the space provided, list what
you should do during each step.

10 Steps	Action Taken
1. Review the Intake Form	_____ _____ _____
2. Perform a Needs Assessment	_____ _____ _____
3. Determine and Rate the Client's Preferences	_____ _____ _____ _____ _____
4. Analyze the Client's Hair	_____ _____ _____
5. Review the Client's Lifestyle	_____ _____

6. Show and Tell

_____

_____

_____

_____

_____

7. Make Recommendations

_____

_____

_____

_____

_____

8. Recommend Color

_____

_____

_____

_____

_____

_____

9. Discuss Upkeep and
   Maintenance

_____

_____

_____

_____

_____

_____

10. Review the Consultation _____

_____

_____

_____

26. A client requests a hairstyle that they have seen on a friend or celebrity that will not suit the client. What should you do?

_____

27. Before making a recommendation to a client about a particular look or style, wait for the client to give you _____ to do so.

28. Which of the following is an example of a client's styling parameter?

_____ a) Hair type   _____ b) Time and ability   _____ c) Face shape

29. Listening to a client and then repeating, in your own words, what you think a client is telling you is called _____.

30. Why do you think it is important to offer a client at least two additional services to complete or improve a style?

_____

_____

_____

_____

_____

_____

31. Explain the three-step plan for making retailing recommendations to a client.

Step 1: _____

Step 2: _____

_____

_____

Step 3: _____

32. At the end of a client consultation, you should not begin the service until you have reviewed everything that you have agreed upon, received the client's _____, and have asked the client for feedback on the consultation process.

33. At the conclusion of the service, what information should you record on the service record card? _____

_____

_____

Handling Communication Barriers

34. Explain why tardy clients create a problem. _____

_____   _____   _____

_____

35. List ways in which tardy clients can be handled so that you do not lose their business or ruin your day's schedule.

a) _____

_____

b) _____

_____

c) _____

_____

d) _____

_____

36. What should you do when a scheduling mix-up occurs?

_____ Do not admit that you or anyone in the salon made a mistake.

_____ Argue with the client about who wrote the appointment down wrong.

_____ Be polite and never argue about who is correct.

_____ Blame the salon receptionist and call the manager.

37. Even though a scheduling mix-up may have the client fuming, you need to stay _____ and move the conversation squarely into resolving the confusion.

38. One guideline for building trust in a dissatisfied client is to try to find out why the client is unhappy by asking for generalities.

_____ True   _____ False

39. Which of the following are appropriate ways of dealing with unhappy clients? (Check all that apply.)

_____ Find out why the client is unhappy.

_____ Do not change what the client dislikes until his or her next visit.

_____ If the problem cannot be fixed, honestly and tactfully explain why.

_____ Argue with the client to make them understand your opinion.

_____ Allow the receptionist to handle the situation so you can move on to your next client.

40. To become a successful stylist, you should only work with clients who share your own age, style, and social background.

_____ True   _____ False

41. What is the best way to decide how to address new clients?

_____ a) Always use their first name.

_____ b) Use the honorific such as "Mrs. Brown" until clients tell you otherwise.

_____ c) Ask clients up front what they would like you to call them.

42. Without both older and younger clients, and ones from different social groups, you will not be able to build a solid client base for future business.

_____ True   _____ False

43. Why should you avoid using slang expressions when speaking with clients?

_____

_____

44. You are performing a consultation on a stylish, younger female client and she uses a slang term to describe how she would like to look. You have no idea what the word means. What should you do next?

_____ a) Agree with whatever she said and hope it is not important.

_____ b) Explain that you have never heard that expression before and ask her to explain what she means.

_____ c) Excuse yourself for a minute and try to find someone who knows what the term means.

45. It is unwise to become a client's counselor, career guide, parental sounding board, or motivational coach.

_____ True   _____ False

46. Which of the following conversation topics are considered neutral and appropriate for use with a client in the salon? (Check all that apply.)

_____ a) A new movie that was just released

_____ b) A scandal involving a local politician

_____ c) Your thoughts on teaching religion in school

_____ d) A new color line the salon is offering

_____ e) Your client's upcoming vacation

47. Think about interactions you have had in the past with other stylists when you have been the *client*. Name three examples of things you have liked about your relationship with a particular stylist. What made the interactions successful?

1) _____

_____

_____

_____

_____

2) _____

_____

_____

_____

_____

3) _____

_____

_____

_____

_____

Guidelines for In-Salon Communication

48. Behaving in a _____ is the first step in making meaningful, in-salon communication a reality.

49. In the salon community, working closely for long hours with your coworkers, it is important to maintain _____ and to remember that the salon is ultimately your place of _____.

50. What points should you keep in mind as you interact and communicate with coworkers?

a) _____

b) _____

c) _____

d) _____

e) _____

f) _____

g) _____

h) _____

51. Describe why you think participating in gossip can be as damaging to you as it is to the object of the gossip.

_____

_____

_____

_____

_____

52. The salon manager is usually the person with the least responsibility regarding the salon's day-to-day operation.

_____ True   _____ False

53. It helps to remember that managers are _____.

54. Staff members should support management and the salon by following the rules and guidelines that are set.

_____ True   _____ False

55. What things should you strive for when dealing with your manager?

a) _____

b) _____

c) _____

d) _____

e) _____

56. What types of salons make it a priority to conduct frequent and thorough employee evaluations? _____

57. It is acceptable for you to request a copy of the form or list of the criteria on which you will be evaluated.

_____ True   _____ False

58. Should you rate yourself in the weeks and months ahead of your evaluation?

_____ Why? _____

_____

_____

59. Why do many professionals never take advantage of the crucial communication opportunity to discuss future advancement with their managers?

_____

60. A self-evaluation demonstrates that you:

_____ do not trust your manager's assessment of your performance.

_____ are planning to look for a new position elsewhere.

_____ are serious about your improvement and growth.

_____ do not think you are doing a good job.

61. At the end of the meeting, you should _____

_____ and for the feedback and guidance they gave you.

62. (W) **ACTIVITY:** Now that you have completed a comprehensive review of the important topic of communicating for success, reflect on what you have learned. Consider and list at least three concepts you have learned in this chapter that relate to your career goals as a cosmetologist. Next to each concept learned, record practical applications that you plan to use to apply those concepts when you become a licensed professional. Prepare a checklist of these behaviors and begin monitoring your desired performance while you are still a student. Use the chart below to list the concepts and intended applications.

Item Number	Concepts	Practical Applications	Rate Performance from Fair to Excellent
1			
2			
3			
4			
5			

INFECTION CONTROL: PRINCIPLES & PRACTICES

Date: _____

Rating: _____

Text Pages: 68–111

why study INFECTION CONTROL: PRINCIPLES AND PRACTICES?

1. Explain in your own words why it is important to study infection control.

_____

_____

_____

_____

_____

_____

_____

Meet the Current Regulations for Health and Safety

2. In regard to regulating the practice of cosmetology, what is the difference between federal agencies and state agencies?

_____

_____

_____

_____

_____

3. What does OSHA stand for?

_____

4. OSHA was created as part of the U. S. Department of Labor (DOL) to _____

_____.

5. What is the purpose of the Hazard Communication Standard (HCS)?

_____

_____

6. Explain why you think OSHA's standards are important to you personally as a cosmetologist.

_____

_____

_____

_____

_____

7. Federal and state laws require manufacturers to supply a Safety Data Sheet (SDS), previously known as Material Safety Data Sheet, only for those products that are potentially hazardous.

_____ True   _____ False

8. List the 16 categories of information contained in a Safety Data Sheet.

_____   _____

_____   _____

_____   _____

_____   _____

_____   _____

_____   _____

_____   _____

_____   _____

9. Federal and state laws require salons to obtain an SDSs from the chemical product manufacturers and/or distributors for each professional product that is used in the salon.

_____ True   _____ False

10. All salon employees must _____ the information included on each SDS and _____ they have done so by _____ a _____ sheet for the product.

11. What does the Environmental Protection Agency (EPA) register?

_____

12. Define the term *disinfectant*. _____

_____

13. Some _____ can be harmful to salon tools and equipment.

14. As a rule of thumb, it is always better to use a tuberculocidal disinfectant when cleaning up a spill in the salon.

_____ True   _____ False

15. By law, a disinfecting product must be used in the manner prescribed on its manufacturer's label and be registered with the EPA.

_____ True   _____ False

16. If you do not follow the instructions for mixing, contact time, and the type of surface the disinfecting product can be used on, you are not complying with federal law.

_____ True   _____ False

17. Why do state regulatory agencies exist? _____

_____

18. List four examples of state regulatory agencies.

1) _____

2) _____

3) _____

4) _____

19. State agency rules are enforced through _____ and investigations of consumer complaints.

20. Explain why it is important for a cosmetologist to understand and follow state laws and rules at all times.

_____

_____

_____

_____

_____

_____

21. What is the difference between laws and rules?

_____

_____

_____

_____

_____

Understand the Principles of Infection

22. The invasion of body tissues by disease-causing pathogens is called

_____.

23. List the four types of microorganisms that are important in the practice of cosmetology.

1) _____

2) _____

3) _____

4) _____

24. Why are the four types of microorganisms listed in the previous question potentially harmful?

_____

25. Use the following terms to complete the sentences below: fungicidal, clean, disinfection, virucidal, bactericidal.

a) _____ refers to something that is capable of destroying viruses.

b) To _____ means to remove all visible debris, dirt, and many disease-causing germs by scrubbing using soap and water or detergent and water.

c) The process of _____ destroys most, but not necessarily all, harmful organisms on environmental surfaces.

d) To destroy a fungi, you would need to use something labeled as a

_____.

e) A product that is _____ is capable of destroying bacteria.

26. Explain why a cosmetologist is obligated to provide safe services in the salon.

_____

_____

_____

27. One-celled microorganisms with both plant and animal characteristics are known as

_____. Where can they exist? _____

_____

_____

28. Most bacteria are _____ which means they are harmless and may perform useful functions.

29. List some of the useful functions of nonpathogenic bacteria.

a) _____

b) _____

c) _____

d) _____

30. Pathogenic bacteria are harmful because they may cause _____ or infection when they invade the body.

31. Match each of the following bacteria with its unique shape.

_____ 1. Cocci   a) Curved lines

_____ 2. Staphylococci   b) Spiral or corkscrew-shaped

_____ 3. Streptococci   c) Short, rod-shaped

_____ 4. Diplococci   d) Round-shaped

_____ 5. Bacilli   e) Grape-like clusters

_____ 6. Spirilla   f) Spherical

32. Pus-forming bacteria that cause abscesses, pustules, and boils are known as

_____.

33. Pus-forming bacteria that cause infections such as strep throat and blood poisoning are known as _____.

34. Diplococci are bacteria that cause diseases such as _____.

35. How do the following bacteria move about?

a) Cocci _____

b) Bacilli _____

c) Spirilla _____

36. A term that means "moving about" is _____ while the term _____ refers to self-movement.

37. Match each term with its correct definition.

_____ 1. Germs

_____ 2. Microorganism

_____ 3. Parasite

_____ 4. Bacteria

_____ 5. Virus

_____ 6. Infection

_____ 7. Toxin

_____ 8. Direct transmission

_____ 9. Indirect transmission

a) Poisonous substances produced by some microorganisms

b) Transmission of body fluids or blood through contact with an intermediate contaminated object

c) One-celled microorganisms having both plant and animal characteristics. Some are harmful and some are harmless

d) Organism of microscopic or submicroscopic size

e) Invasion of body tissues by disease-causing pathogens

f) Transmission of blood or body fluids through touching, kissing, coughing, sneezing, and talking

g) An organism that grows, feeds, and shelters on or in another organism while contributing nothing to the survival of that organism

h) Synonym for any disease-producing organism

i) A submicroscopic particle that infects and resides in the cells of a biological organism

38. Unscramble these words and use them to complete the sentences below.

briateac   sopotparlm   crdoeupre   cniatvie

_____ generally consist of an outer cell wall containing a liquid called _____. They grow and _____. The life cycle of bacteria is made up of two distinct phases: the active stage and the _____ or spore-forming stage.

39. During the active stage, bacteria:

_____ a) change color

_____ b) die

_____ c) grow and reproduce

_____ d) dry out

40. The division of a bacteria cell is called _____. The cells that are formed are called _____.

41. What type of conditions do bacteria require to multiply?

_____ a) Cool and dark   _____ c) Dark and dry

_____ b) Warm and clean   _____ d) Warm, dark, and damp

42. What happens to bacteria in favorable conditions? _____
What happens in unfavorable conditions?

_____

43. Why do certain bacteria, such as tetanus and botulism, coat themselves with wax-like outer shells?

_____

44. What happens to bacteria when favorable conditions are restored?

_____

45. There can be no bacterial infection without the presence of

_____.

46. _____ is the body's reaction to injury, irritation, or infection;
it may be characterized by _____, _____,
_____, and _____.

47. What is pus?

_____

48. A local infection is one that is _____ to a particular part of the body.

49. Give an example of a local infection. _____

50. Staphylococci are among the most common human bacteria and are more frequently spread through skin-to-skin contact or through _____

_____.

51. An example of a staph infection is MRSA, which stands for _____

_____.

52. Historically, MRSA occurred most frequently in people who have _____
immune systems or who had undergone _____ procedures.

53. MRSA initially appears as a skin infection such as _____.

54. It is possible for a client to have a staph infection without knowing it.

_____ True   _____ False

55. A disease that spreads from one person to another by contact is said to be contagious or _____.

56. List the more common contagious diseases that will prevent a cosmetologist from servicing a client. _____

_____

57. List 12 ways contagious diseases are commonly spread.

1) _____

2) _____

3) _____

4) _____

5) _____

6) _____

7) _____

8) _____

9) _____

10) _____

11) _____

12) _____

58. What are two differences between bacteria and viruses?

1) _____

_____

_____

2) _____

_____

_____

59. Vaccinations prevent viruses from growing in the body, but are not available for all viruses.

_____ True   _____ False

60. The human papilloma virus (HPV) can infect the bottoms of the _____.

61. A client who shows signs of an HPV infection should not receive a _____ service.

62. Disease-causing microorganisms that are carried in the body by blood or body fluids are called _____.

63. List nine ways bloodborne pathogens can be spread inside the salon.

1) _____

2) _____

3) _____

4) _____

5) _____

6) _____

7) _____

8) _____

9) _____

64. It is against the law for a cosmetologist to _____, even if the client insists.

65. Cutting hardened tissue and removing a callus are both considered _____.

66. What are the three types of hepatitis that are of concern in the salon? _____

67. Which of the three types of hepatitis is the most difficult to kill on a surface? _____

68. What does HIV stand for? _____

69. What does AIDS stand for? _____
What is AIDS? _____

70. Name some ways in which HIV is not spread. _____

_____

71. _____, which include molds, mildews, and yeasts, can cause _____ diseases such as ringworm.

72. Although it affects plants or grows on inanimate objects, _____ does not cause human infections in the salon.

73. _____ is a superficial fungal infection caused by a variety of dermatophytes. What does it affect? _____ _____ Whom does it mostly affect? _____

74. List the two steps that should be followed to clean and disinfect clipper blades effectively.

1) _____

2) _____

75. Nail infections can be spread by using ____ _____ implements or by not properly _____ the surface of the natural nail before applying an enhancement.

76. A _____ nail infection is more common on the feet than on the hands.

77. _____ nail infections commonly occur on both the hands and the feet.

78. Which of the following is the most frequently encountered infection on the foot resulting from nail services?

_____ a) Tinea barbae   _____ b) Tinea pedis   _____ c) Tinea capitis

79. _____ are organisms that grow, feed, and shelter on or in another _____, referred to as a host, while contributing _____ to the survival of that organism.

80. Name three external parasites that affect the human skin.

1) _____

2) _____

3) _____

81. Match each of the following terms with its definition.

_____ 1. Immunity   a) Both inherited and developed through healthy living

_____ 2. Natural immunity   b) Ability to overcome disease through inoculation or exposure to natural allergens like pollen

_____ 3. Acquired immunity   c) The body's ability to destroy, resist, and recognize infection

Prevent the Spread of Disease

82. Proper _____ can prevent the spread of disease caused by exposure to potentially infectious material on an item's surface.

83. When proper cleaning and then _____ with an appropriate _____ disinfectant occur, virtually all pathogens of concern in the salon can be effectively eliminated.

84. _____, which is the process that destroys all microbial life, is an infection-control method that can be used, but it is very rarely mandated.

85. The Centers for Disease Control and Prevention (CDC) requires that autoclaves be tested _____ to ensure they are properly sterilizing implements.

86. Define the term decontamination. _____

_____

_____

87. Putting antiseptics on your skin, or just washing your hands with soap and water, will reduce the number of pathogens on your hands, but it does not _____

_____.

88. When cleaning, you must remove all _____ from tools, implements, and equipment by washing with liquid soap and warm water and by using a clean and _____ to scrub any grooved or hinged portions of the item.

89. Three ways to clean tools and implements include washing and scrubbing with soap and water, using an ultraviolet unit, and using a cleaning solvent.

_____ True   _____ False

90. An autoclave that incorporates heat and pressure is typically required for effective _____.

91. What is the accepted method for testing an autoclave to ensure it is properly sterilizing implements? _____.

92. The vast majority of pathogens and contaminants can be removed from the surfaces of tools and implements through proper cleaning.

_____ True   _____ False

93. If you are in a hurry to get to your next client, it is acceptable to use a disinfectant on an instrument and skip the step of cleaning it first.

_____ True   _____ False

94. Disinfectants are products that destroy most _____, excluding spores, on surfaces.

95. Explain how sterilization is different from disinfection.

_____

_____

_____

_____

96. Explain why disinfectants should not be used on human skin, hair, or nails.

_____

_____

_____

_____

97. Disinfectants must be registered by the _____.

_____ CDC   _____ FDA   _____ EPA

98. What does it mean if a disinfectant has the word *concentrate* on its label?

_____ It must be diluted as instructed before using.

_____ It is ready to use right out of the container.

_____ It is less potent than other types of disinfectants.

99. Define the term *contact time*.

_____

_____

100. Define efficacy as applied to disinfectant terms.

_____

_____

101. When compared to a hospital, a salon has a _____ infection risk.

_____ higher   _____ lower

102. What are four things a cosmetologist should know about accelerated hydrogen peroxide (AHP)?

1) _____

2) _____

3) _____

4) _____

103. Explain why you need to remove all dirt and other matter you can see on tools and implements before immersing them in disinfectant solution.

_____

_____

_____

104. The label on a disinfectant product states "complete immersion." Explain what this means.

_____

_____

_____

105. To disinfect large surfaces such as tabletops, carefully apply the disinfectant onto the pre-cleaned surface, or use a disinfectant spray and allow it to remain wet for 5 minutes.

_____ True   _____ False

106. _____, also known as quats, are effective disinfectants for salon use, when properly used in the salon.

107. List six disadvantages of phenolic disinfectants.

1) _____

2) _____

3) _____

4) _____

5) _____

6) _____

108. Any type of household bleach may be used as an effective disinfectant.

_____ True   _____ False

109. Name five disadvantages of using bleach as a disinfectant.

1) _____

2) _____

3) _____

4) _____

5) _____

110. Identify each of the following items used in a salon as either multiuse or single-use.

Nippers _____

Cotton balls _____

Permanent wave rods _____

Combs _____

Shears _____

Nail files _____

Wooden sticks _____

111. Currently, no states require salons to clean and disinfect their multiuse tools and implements.

_____ True   _____ False

112. According to state rules, how often should multiuse tools and equipment be cleaned and then disinfected? _____

113. Why is it good practice to keep a logbook of all equipment usage, cleaning, disinfecting, testing, and maintenance?

_____

_____

_____

_____

114. In the salon, how should soiled linens and towels be stored until they can be properly laundered?

_____

_____

_____

115. Mix all disinfectants according to the manufacturer's directions, always adding water to the disinfectant.

_____ True   _____ False

116. A water sanitizer does not properly clean or disinfect equipment.

_____ True   _____ False

117. The true benefit of hand washing comes from the _____ created by the _____ that can "pull" pathogens off the skin surface.

118. (W) **ACTIVITY:** Using the following chart as a template, research the various disinfectant products used in the school and in your home. (*Answers will vary based on the disinfectants the students find at home and in the school.*)

Disinfectant	Key Ingredients	Description of How It is Used	List Required Safety Precautions
Example: Clorox Clean-Up	Sodium Hypochlorite; Dimethicone/Silica /PEG Disterate Antifoam	Spray product 4–6 inches from surface until thoroughly wet. Let stand 30 seconds. Rinse or wipe clean.	Use only in well-ventilated areas. Avoid contact with clothes, fabric, wood, rubber, painted, and paper surfaces.

Follow Standard Precautions to Protect You and Your Clients

119. What are Standard Precautions?

_____

_____

_____

120. Explain why strict infection control practices should be followed for every client.

_____

_____

_____

_____

121. Contact with nonintact skin, blood, body fluid, and/or other potentially infectious materials that is the result of the performance of an employee's duties is known as

_____ .

List Your Professional Responsibilities

122. _____ should be a part of the normal routine for you and your coworkers so the salon and staff project a professional image.

123. How often should you sweep hair off the floor of the salon?

_____ a) After every client

_____ b) Once a day

_____ c) As part of the closing routine

124. What are the benefits of keeping trash in a covered waste receptacle?

_____

125. To maintain a professional image, try to avoid touching your _____, _____, or _____ during client services.

126. Where should clean and disinfected tools be stored?

_____

127. How often should fans, ventilation systems, and humidifiers be cleaned?

_____

128. What is a way to ensure proper air quality in the salon?

_____

6 GENERAL ANATOMY & PHYSIOLOGY

Date: _____

Rating: _____

Text Pages: 112–151

why study ANATOMY AND PHYSIOLOGY?

1. List the reasons a cosmetologist studies anatomy and physiology.

a) _____

_____

_____

b) _____

_____

_____

_____

c) _____

_____

_____

Why Anatomy and Physiology Are Important to You

2. Before you begin this chapter, think about the areas of anatomy and physiology with which you are already familiar with from past studies or experiences. As you think about your career as a cosmetologist, which body systems do you think will be most important for you to understand well?

_____

_____

_____

3. As a cosmetologist, you should have an overall knowledge of human anatomy, however, cosmetology is primarily limited to _____

_____.

4. The study of human body structures that can be seen with the naked eye and how the body parts are organized is called _____.

5. _____ is the study of the functions and activities performed by the body's structures.

Describe Cells

6. The basic unit of all living things, from bacteria to plants to animals, including human beings is the _____.

7. Identify the parts of the cell in the following illustration.

8. The cells of all living things are composed of a substance called _____, a colorless, jelly-like substance found inside cells in which food elements such as proteins, fats, carbohydrates, mineral salts, and water are present.

9. Match each of the following terms with its definition.

_____ 1. Mitosis   a) The dense, active protoplasm found in the center of the cell

_____ 2. Nucleus   b) The watery fluid that surrounds the nucleus of the cell and is needed for growth, reproduction, and self-repair

_____ 3. Cytoplasm   c) The process of cell reproduction of human tissues that occurs when the cell divides into two identical cells

_____ 4. Cell membrane   d) The part of the cell that encloses the protoplasm and permits soluble substances to enter and leave the cell

10. Cells have the ability to reproduce, thus providing new cells for the growth and replacement of worn or injured ones.

_____ True   _____ False

11. Mitosis is the usual process of cell reproduction of human tissues that occurs when the cell divides into two identical cells called _____.

12. For cells to grow and reproduce, conditions must be _____, which include:

a) _____

b) _____

c) _____

Define Tissues

13. A collection of similar cells that perform a particular function are _____. Each kind has a specific function and can be recognized by its _____ appearance.

14. How many types of tissue are there in the body? _____

15. _____ tissue is a protective covering on body surfaces.

_____ a) Connective   _____ d) Nerve

_____ b) Epithelial   _____ e) Adipose

_____ c) Muscle

16. _____ tissue contracts and moves the various parts of the body.

_____ a) Connective   _____ d) Nerve

_____ b) Epithelial   _____ e) Adipose

_____ c) Muscle

17. _____ tissue is fibrous tissue that binds together, protects, and supports the various parts of the body.

_____ a) Connective   _____ d) Nerve

_____ b) Epithelial   _____ e) Adipose

_____ c) Muscle

18. Tissues that give smoothness and contour to the body while protecting internal organs and insulating the body are _____.

_____ a) connective   _____ d) nerve

_____ b) epithelial   _____ e) adipose

_____ c) muscle

19. _____ tissues carry messages to and from the brain and control and coordinate all bodily functions.

_____ a) Connective   _____ d) Nerve

_____ b) Epithelial   _____ e) Adipose

_____ c) Muscle

20. List examples of connective tissue. _____

_____

21. List examples of epithelial tissue. _____

_____

22. Nerve tissue is composed of special cells known as _____ that make up the nerves, brain, and spinal cord.

Name the Organs and Body Systems

23. Structures composed of specialized tissues designed to perform specific functions in plants and animals are _____.

24. _____ are groups of body organs acting together to perform one or more functions. There are _____ major systems.

25. Give the functions of the following systems.

a) Circulatory: _____

_____

_____

b) Digestive: _____

_____

_____

c) Endocrine: _____

_____

_____

d) Excretory: _____

_____

_____

e) Integumentary: _____

_____

_____

f) Immune (lymphatic): _____

_____

_____

g) Muscular: _____

_____

_____

h) Nervous: _____

_____

_____

i) Reproductive: _____

_____

_____

j) Respiratory: _____

_____

_____

k) Skeletal: _____

_____

_____

Review the Skeletal System

26. The skeletal system forms the physical foundation of the body and is composed of _____ bones that vary in size and shape and are connected by _____ and _____ joints.

27. Other than bone, what is the hardest tissue in the body? _____

_____

28. List the five primary functions of the skeletal system.

1) _____

_____

2) _____

_____

3) _____

_____

4) _____

_____

5) _____

_____

29. A _____ is the connection between two or more bones of the skeleton.

30. The two types of joints are _____. What are some examples of each type? _____

_____

31. The skull is divided into two parts: the _____, an oval, bony case that protects the brain, and the _____, the framework of the face that is composed of _____ bones.

32. The cranium is made up of:

_____ a) eight bones.   _____ c) two bones.

_____ b) ten bones.   _____ d) fourteen bones.

33. Match each of the following bones of the cranium with its description.

_____ 1. Parietal   a) Forms the forehead

_____ 2. Occipital   b) Hindmost bone of the skull

_____ 3. Frontal   c) Form the sides of the head in the ear region

_____ 4. Temporal   d) Form the sides and top of the cranium

_____ 5. Ethmoid   e) Join all the bones of the cranium together

_____ 6. Sphenoid   f) Form part of the nasal cavities

34. Match each of the following bones of the face with its description.

_____ 1. Nasal   a) Small, thin bones located at the front inner wall

_____ 2. Lacrimal   b) Lower jawbone, largest and strongest bone of
                                the face

_____ 3. Zygomatic   c) Form the bridge of the nose

_____ 4. Maxillae   d) Bones of the upper jaw

_____ 5. Mandible   e) Form the prominence of the cheeks

35. Match each of the following bones of the neck, chest, shoulder, and back with its description.

_____ 1. Hyoid   a) U-shaped bone at the base of the tongue

_____ 2. Cervical vertebrae b) The chest; elastic, bony cage

_____ 3. Thorax   c) Shoulder blade

_____ 4. Ribs   d) Collarbone

_____ 5. Scapula   e) Breastbone

_____ 6. Sternum   f) Twelve pairs of bones forming the wall of the thorax

_____ 7. Clavicle   g) Seven bones of the top part of the vertebral column

36. The smaller bone in the forearm on the same side as the thumb is the:

_____ a) humerus.   _____ c) carpus.

_____ b) radius.   _____ d) ulna.

37. The uppermost and largest bone in the arm is the:

_____ a) humerus.   _____ c) carpus.

_____ b) radius.   _____ d) ulna.

38. Another name for the wrist, a flexible joint composed of a group of eight small, irregular bones held together by ligaments, is the _____.

39. The inner and larger bone in the forearm, which is attached to the wrist and located on the side of the little finger, is the _____.

40. The _____ are the bones of the palm of the hand, and the phalanges are the bones of the fingers and toes, also called _____.

41. Match each of the following terms with its description.

_____ 1. Femur   a) Accessory bone; forms the kneecap joint

_____ 2. Tibia   b) Heavy, long bone; forms the leg above the knee

_____ 3. Fibula   c) Smaller of the two bones that form the leg below the knee

_____ 4. Patella   d) Ankle bone; bone of the ankle joint

_____ 5. Talus   e) Larger of two bones that form the leg below the knee

42. The foot is made up of _____ bones, subdivided into three categories:

1) _____

2) _____

3) _____

43. 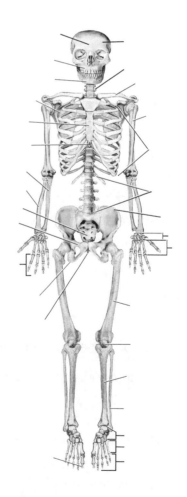 **ACTIVITY:** Working alone or with a partner, use large sheets of paper such as newsprint, flip chart, or party table paper, and draw all the major bones of the human skeleton. Cut each major bone out separately and use colored markers to label each bone. Use a single-hole punch and paperclips to assemble the parts into a life-sized skeleton that can be hung from a hook or hanger.

Review the Muscular System

44. Define the muscular system. _____

_____

_____

45. Muscles are _____ that have the ability to stretch and contract according to demands of the body's movements.

46. Name the three parts of the muscle and define each part.

1) _____

2) _____

3) _____

47. In which direction is pressure applied to the muscle during massage?

_____

48. List seven ways in which muscular tissue can be stimulated.

1) _____

2) _____

3) _____

4) _____

5) _____

6) _____

7) _____

49. The broad muscle that covers the top of the skull is the _____.
It consists of two parts: the _____ and the
_____.

50. The muscle that draws the scalp backward is the _____.

51. The _____ muscle of the scalp raises the eyebrows, draws the scalp forward, and causes wrinkles across the forehead.

52. What tendon connects the occipitalis and the frontalis muscles?

_____

53. The broad muscle extending from the chest and shoulder muscles to the side of the chin is the _____. What is its responsibility? _____

_____

54. Which muscle of the neck lowers and rotates the head?

_____

55. The muscle located beneath the frontalis and orbicularis oculi muscle that draws the eyebrow down and wrinkles the forehead vertically is the:

_____ a) corrugator.   _____ c) orbicularis oris.

_____ b) orbicularis oculi.   _____ d) procerus.

56. The muscle that covers the bridge of the nose, lowers the eyebrows, and causes wrinkles across the bridge of the nose is the:

_____ a) corrugator.   _____ c) orbicularis oris.

_____ b) orbicularis oculi.   _____ d) procerus.

57. The ring muscle of the eye socket, enabling you to close your eyes, is the:

_____ a) corrugator.   _____ c) orbicularis oris.

_____ b) orbicularis oculi.   _____ d) procerus.

58. Match each of the following muscles of the mouth with its description.

_____ 1. Buccinator

a) Muscle that elevates the lower lip and raises and wrinkles the skin of the chin

_____ 2. Depressor labii inferioris

b) Muscles on both sides of the face that extend from the zygomatic bone to the angle of the mouth; pull the mouth upward and backward

_____ 3. Levator anguli oris

c) Thin, flat muscle of the cheek between the upper and lower jaw that compresses the cheeks and expels air between the lips

_____ 4. Levator labii superioris

d) Muscle that raises the angle of the mouth and draws it inward

_____ 5. Mentalis

e) Muscle of the mouth that draws the corner of the mouth out and back

_____ 6. Orbicularis oris

f) Muscle extending alongside the chin that pulls down the corner of the mouth

_____ 7. Risorius

g) Muscle surrounding the lower lip; lowers the lip and draws it to one side

_____ 8. Triangularis

h) Flat band of muscle around the upper and lower lips that compresses, contracts, puckers, and wrinkles the lips

_____ 9. Zygomaticus major   i) Muscle surrounding the upper lip; elevates the upper lip and dilates the nostrils

_____ 10. Zygomaticus minor   j) Muscles on both sides of the face that extend from the zygomatic bone to the upper lips; pull the upper lip backward, upward, and outward

59. The large, flat, triangular muscle covering the lower back is the:

_____ a) pectoralis major.   _____ c) latissimus dorsi.

_____ b) serratus anterior.   _____ d) trapezius.

60. The muscle that covers the back of the neck and the upper and middle region of the back and rotates and controls the swinging movements of the arm is the:

_____ a) pectoralis major.   _____ c) latissimus dorsi.

_____ b) serratus anterior.   _____ d) trapezius.

61. The muscles of the chest that assist the swinging movements of the arm are the:

_____ a) pectoralis major.   _____ c) latissimus dorsi.

_____ b) serratus anterior.   _____ d) trapezius.

62. The muscle of the chest that assists in breathing and in raising the arm is the:

_____ a) pectoralis major.   _____ c) latissimus dorsi.

_____ b) serratus anterior.   _____ d) trapezius.

63. What are the three principal muscles of the shoulders and upper arms?

_____

64. Match each of the following muscles with its description.

_____ 1. Bicep   a) Muscles that straighten the wrist, hand, and fingers to form a straight line

_____ 2. Deltoid   b) Muscle that produces the contour of the front and inner side of the upper arm; lifts the forearm and flexes the elbow

_____ 3. Triceps   c) Muscle that turns the hand inward so that the palm faces downward

_____ 4. Extensor   d) Muscle of the forearm that rotates the radius outward and the palm upward

_____ 5. Flexor   e) Large, triangular muscle covering the shoulder joint that allows the arm to extend outward and to the side of the body

_____ 6. Pronator   f) Extensor muscle of the wrist involved in flexing the wrist

_____ 7. Supinator   g) Large muscle that covers the entire back of the upper arm and extends the forearm

65. What is the difference between the abductor and adductor muscles?

_____

_____

_____

66. The muscle that bends the foot up and extends the toes is the:

_____ a) peroneus brevis.   _____ c) peroneus longus.

_____ b) tibialis anterior.   _____ d) extensor digitorum longus.

67. The muscle that covers the front of the shin and bends the foot upward and inward is the:

_____ a) peroneus brevis.   _____ c) peroneus longus.

_____ b) tibialis anterior.   _____ d) extensor digitorum longus.

68. The muscle that covers the outer side of the calf and inverts the foot and turns it outward is the:

_____ a) peroneus brevis.   _____ c) peroneus longus.

_____ b) tibialis anterior.   _____ d) extensor digitorum longus.

69. The muscle that originates at the upper portion of the fibula and bends the foot down is the:

_____ a) gastrocnemius.   _____ c) peroneus brevis.

_____ b) soleus.   _____ d) peroneus longus.

70. The muscle attached to the lower rear surface of the heel that pulls the foot down is the:

_____ a) gastrocnemius.   _____ c) peroneus brevis.

_____ b) soleus.   _____ d) peroneus longus.

71. Name the muscles of the feet.

a) _____

b) _____

c) _____

d) _____

Review the Nervous System

72. The system that is an exceptionally well-organized and is responsible for controlling and coordinating all other systems of the body and makes them work harmoniously and efficiently is the _____.

73. What is the central nervous system composed of?

_____

74. _____ is the scientific study of the structure, function, and pathology of the nervous system.

75. Why is it important for a cosmetologist to understand how the nervous system works?

_____

_____

76. List the three main subdivisions of the nervous system.

1) _____

2) _____

3) _____

77. Name the subdivision of the nervous system identified by each of the following descriptions.

_____ System of nerves that connects the outer parts of the body to the central nervous system

_____ Consists of the brain, spinal cord, spinal nerves, and cranial nerves

_____ Controls the involuntary muscles

_____ Regulates the action of the smooth muscles, glands, blood vessels, heart, and breath

_____ Controls consciousness and many mental activities, functions of the five senses, and voluntary muscle actions

_____ Carries impulses, or messages, to and from the central nervous system

78. The _____ is the largest and most complex organization of nerve tissue, and it controls sensation; muscles; activity of _____; and the power to think, sense, and feel.

79. The portion of the central nervous system that originates in the brain and extends down to the lower extremity of the trunk, and is protected by the spinal column is the _____. How many pairs of spinal nerves extend from it? _____

80. The whitish cords made up of bundles of nerve fibers, held together by connective tissue, through which impulses are transmitted are _____. Where do they have their origin? _____

81. There are _____ types of nerves: _____, which carry impulses or messages from the sense organs to the brain, and _____, which carry impulses from the brain to the muscles or glands.

82. The two types of nerves are also known as _____ nerves and _____ nerves.

83. The sensations of touch, cold, heat, sight, sound, taste, smell, pain, and pressure are experienced by the _____ nerves.

84. How does information about different sensations reach the brain?

_____

_____

_____

_____

85. The impulses that produce movement are transmitted by the _____ nerves.

86. What is a reflex and how does it work?

_____

_____

_____

_____

87. Which of the cranial nerves is the largest? _____ List the two additional names for this nerve. _____ What is the purpose of this nerve? _____

_____

_____

88. List the three branches of the fifth cranial nerve and their function.

1) _____ _____

_____

_____

_____

2) _____ _____

_____

_____

_____

3) _____ _____

_____

_____

_____

89. The chief motor nerve of the face is the _____ cranial nerve.

90. List the most important branches of the facial nerve.

a) _____

b) _____

c) _____

d) _____

e) _____

f) _____

91. Which nerve controls the motion of the neck and shoulder muscles and is affected during facials, primarily when giving a massage to your client?

_____

92. The principal nerves of the arm and hand are the _____,

_____, _____, and the _____.

93. Identify the nerves of the arm and hand in the illustration.

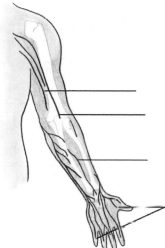

94. The nerve that subdivides and supplies impulses to the knee; the muscles of the calf; the skin of the leg; and the sole, heel, and underside of the toes is the

_____.

95. Match each of the following terms with its definition.

_____ 1. Common peroneal nerve

a) Extends down the leg, just under the skin, supplying impulses to the muscles and the skin of the leg

_____ 2. Deep peroneal nerve

b) Extends from behind the knee to wind around the head of the fibula to the front of the leg

_____ 3. Superficial peroneal nerve

c) Extends down to the front of the leg, behind the muscles; supplies impulses to these muscles and to the muscles and skin on top of the foot and adjacent sides of the first and second toes

96. Which nerve supplies impulses to the skin on the outer side and back of the foot and leg?

_____ a) Saphenous   _____ c) Dorsal

_____ b) Sural   _____ d) Tibial

97. Which nerve extends up from the toes and foot, just under the skin, supplying impulses to the toes, foot, and muscles of the skin of the leg?

_____ a) Saphenous   _____ c) Dorsal

_____ b) Sural   _____ d) Tibial

Review the Circulatory System

98. The circulatory system, also known as the _____ or
_____ system, controls the steady circulation of the blood through the
body by means of the heart and blood vessels. It consists of the _____
_____.

99. The purpose of the circulatory system is to _____
_____.

100. Which of the following is referred to as the body's pump?

_____ a) Cells   _____ c) Heart

_____ b) Lungs   _____ d) Veins

101. The blood is in constant and continuous circulation from the time that it leaves the
heart, is distributed throughout the body to deliver _____, and then
returns to the heart to be sent to the lungs and replenished with oxygen.

102. Explain how pulmonary and systemic circulation work.

_____

_____

_____

_____

_____

_____

103. The types of blood vessels important to a cosmetologist are _____,
_____, _____, _____, and
_____.

104. Match each of the following terms with its description.

_____ 1. Arteries   a) Tiny, thin-walled blood vessels that connect the smaller
                             arteries to venules

_____ 2. Capillaries   b) Thin-walled blood vessels that are less elastic than arteries

_____ 3. Veins   c) Thick-walled, muscular, flexible tubes that carry
                             oxygenated blood away from the heart to the arterioles

_____ 4. Venules   d) Small arteries that deliver blood to capillaries

_____ 5. Arterioles   e) Small vessels that connect the capillaries to the veins

105. What is blood? _____

106. There are approximately _____ pints of blood in the human body. Blood is approximately _____ water.

107. What five critical functions does blood perform?

1) _____

_____

2) _____

_____

3) _____

_____

4) _____

_____

5) _____

_____

108. The _____ arteries are the main arteries that supply blood to the head, face, and neck, and they are located on both sides of the neck.

109. The internal carotid artery supplies blood to the _____

_____.

110. The external carotid artery supplies blood to the _____

_____.

111. The artery that supplies blood to the lower region of the face, mouth, and nose is the:

_____ a) facial artery.   _____ c) superficial temporal artery.

_____ b) angular artery.   _____ d) superior labial artery.

112. The artery that supplies blood to the upper lip and region of the nose is the:

_____ a) facial artery.   _____ c) superficial temporal artery.

_____ b) angular artery.   _____ d) superior labial artery.

113. The artery that supplies blood to the skin and masseter muscle is the:

_____ a) parietal artery.   _____ c) middle temporal artery.

_____ b) transverse facial artery.   _____ d) anterior auricular artery.

114. The _____ and _____ arteries are the main blood supply of the arms and hands.

115. Identify the arteries of the arm and hand in the following illustration:

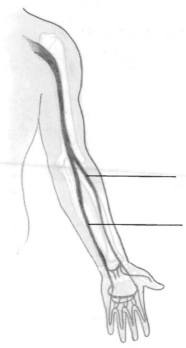

116. The popliteal artery divides into two separate arteries; one of these is called the:

_____ a) parietal artery.   _____ c) anterior tibial artery.

_____ b) transverse facial artery.   _____ d) anterior auricular artery.

Review the Lymphatic/Immune System

117. The lymphatic/immune system is closely related to the _____ system and consists of the _____

_____.

118. What is the purpose of the lymphatic/immune system?

_____

_____

_____

119. List the primary functions of the lymphatic/immune system.

a) _____

_____

b) _____

_____

c) _____

_____

d) _____

_____

Review the Integumentary System

120. The _____ consists of the skin and its accessory organs, such as the _____, _____,

_____, and _____.

121. The integumentary system serves as a water-resistant, _____ and helps regulate the body's temperature.

Review the Endocrine System

122. The endocrine system is a group of specialized glands that affect:

a) _____

b) _____

c) _____

d) _____

123. What are glands? _____

_____

124. Name the two main types of glands and their functions.

1) _____

_____

2) _____

_____

125. What are hormones? _____

_____

126. Give three examples of hormones.

1) _____

2) _____

3) _____

127. The thyroid gland plays a role in which of the following?

        a) Sexual development   _____ c) Metabolism

        b) Blood pressure   _____ d) Digesting carbohydrates

128. The pituitary gland affects almost every _____ of the body.

129. The pineal gland plays a major role in which of the following?

        a) Sexual development   _____ c) Breast-milk production

        b) Blood pressure   _____ d) Sexual organ function

Review the Reproductive System

130. The organs on the female reproductive system include the _____

_____.

131. The organs on the male reproductive system include the _____

_____.

132. What are some unwanted results that may be caused by fluctuating female or male hormones? _____

_____

CHAPTER 7

SKIN STRUCTURE, GROWTH, & NUTRITION

Date: _____

Rating: _____

Text Pages: 152–169

why study SKIN STRUCTURE, GROWTH, AND NUTRITION?

1. Clients with adverse conditions, including skin diseases, inflamed skin, and infectious skin disorders should be referred to a medical professional for treatment.

   _____ True   _____ False

2. Describe in your own words why you think it is necessary for a cosmetologist to stay on top of changes in skin care.

   _____

   _____

   _____

   _____

   _____

   _____

   _____

   _____

Know the Anatomy of the Skin

3. The medical branch of science that deals with the study of skin and its nature, structure, functions, diseases, and treatment is called _____

   _____.

4. A _____ is a physician who specializes in diseases and disorders of the skin, hair, and nails.

5. Some skin symptoms may be a sign of internal _____.

6. By law, in all states cosmetologists may clean skin, preserve the health of skin, and beautify skin.

   _____ True   _____ False

7. An _____ specializes in the cleansing, beautification, and preservation of the health of skin on the entire body, including the face and neck.

8. This professional may diagnose an abnormal skin condition:

   _____ esthetician.   _____ cosmetologist.   _____ nutritionist.   _____ dermatologist.

9. The skin is the largest organ of the body.

   _____ True   _____ False

10. The skin is the only natural barrier between our bodies and the environment and protects the network of:

    a) _____

    b) _____

    c) _____

    d) _____

    e) _____

11. Please describe the ideal appearance of healthy skin.

    _____

    _____

12. List the appendages of the skin.

    a) _____

    b) _____

    c) _____

    d) _____

13. Explain how a callus forms and state an example of how you think one may occur.

    _____

    _____

    _____

    _____

14. When is it appropriate to completely remove a callus in the salon?

_____

_____

_____

15. Explain the difference between the skin of the scalp and the skin elsewhere on the human body.

_____

_____

_____

16. The skin is composed of two main divisions: the _____ and the _____ .

17. Identify the layers of the skin illustrated below:

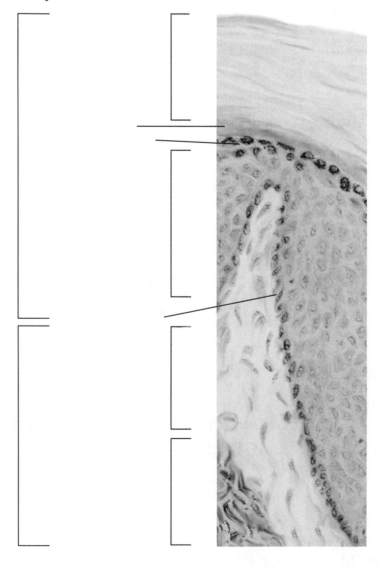

18. The _____ is the outermost and _____
    layer of the skin.

19. Name the five layers that make up the epidermis.

    1) _____

    2) _____

    3) _____

    4) _____

    5) _____

20. The thinnest skin is found under or around the _____, and the thickest
    skin is found on the _____.

21. The basal cell layer is also referred to as the _____ and is the
    deepest layer of the epidermis. It is the _____ of the epidermis
    that produces new epidermal skin cells and is responsible for the growth of the

    _____.

22. The basal cell layer contains special cells called _____, which produce
    the dark skin pigment called _____.

23. The _____, also referred to as the stratum spinosum, is the layer where
    the process of skin cell shedding begins.

24. The stratum granulosum, or _____, is composed of cells that look like
    granules and are filled with keratin. The cells die as they are pushed to the surface to
    replace _____ that are shed from the stratum corneum.

25. The _____ is the clear, transparent layer under the _____
    and consists of small cells through which light can pass.

26. Which layer of the skin is cared for by salon products and services?

    _____ Stratum corneum   _____ Stratum spinosum

    _____ Stratum lucidum   _____ Stratum germinativum

27. The highly sensitive dermis layer of connective tissue is about _____
    times thicker than the epidermis.

28. The _____ is the underlying or inner layer of the skin and is made up of
    two layers: the _____ and the _____.

29. Describe what causes goose bumps or goose flesh.

_____

_____

_____

30. Which layer is the outer layer of the dermis, located directly beneath the epidermis?

_____

31. Which layer is the deeper layer of the dermis that supplies the skin with all of its oxygen and nutrients? _____

32. The reticular layer contains the following structures within its network:

a) _____

b) _____

c) _____

d) _____

e) _____

f) _____

g) _____

h) _____

33. Where is the subcutaneous tissue found? _____

34. The subcutaneous tissue is also called _____ or _____ tissue and varies in thickness according to the _____, _____, and _____.

35. What are the functions of fatty tissue?

_____

_____

36. _____ delivers nutrients and oxygen to the skin. _____, the clear fluids of the body that bathe the skin cells, _____ and _____ and have immune functions that help protect the skin and body against diseases.

37. The skin contains the surface endings of the following nerve fibers:

a) _____

b) _____

c) _____

38. _____ nerve fibers react to heat, cold, touch, pressure, and pain.

39. _____ nerve fibers are distributed to the arrector pili muscles attached to the hair follicles.

40. Which nerve fibers are part of the autonomic nervous system, regulate the excretion of perspiration from the sudoriferous glands, and control the flow of sebum to the surface of the skin? _____

41. The nerve endings that provide the body with the sense of touch, pain, heat, cold, and pressure are housed in the _____ layer of the dermis.

42. Complex sensations, such as _____, seem to depend on the sensitivity of a combination of the nerve endings found in the papillary layer of the dermis.

43. The color of the skin depends primarily on _____, which are tiny grains of pigment that are produced by melanocytes and then deposited into cells in the _____ of the epidermis and papillary layers of the dermis.

44. Name and describe the two types of melanin.

    1) _____

    2) _____

45. The color of the skin is a _____ trait, and your _____ determine the amount and type of pigment produced in an individual.

46. Why do you need to use a broad spectrum sunscreen if melanin helps protect your body from the sun?

    _____

    _____

    _____

    _____

    _____

    _____

47. The skin gets its strength, form, and flexibility from two specific structures found in the dermis:

    1) _____   2) _____

48. What are some causes of wrinkles and sagging skin?

_____

_____

49. According to the majority of scientists, most signs of skin aging are caused by

_____.

50. Using a daily broad spectrum sunscreen with an SPF of 15 or higher, maintaining a moisturizing skincare regimen, and keeping the skin _____will slow the weakening of collagen and elastin fibers and help skin look young longer.

51. The skin contains two types of duct glands, _____ _____ and

_____ _____.

52. In addition to detoxifying the body by excreting salt and unwanted chemicals, the sudoriferous glands excrete:

_____ a) fragrance.   _____ c) oil.

_____ b) water.   _____ d) perspiration.

53. The sweat glands regulate _____ and help eliminate

_____ _____ from the body. They are found on practically all parts of the body, but are more numerous on the _____

_____.

54. The excretion of sweat is controlled by the _____, and normally one to two pints of salt-containing liquids are eliminated daily through _____ in the skin.

55. The sebaceous or oil glands of the skin are connected to the _____. These glands secrete _____, a fatty or oily substance.

56. Sebaceous glands are not found on the:

_____ a) scalp.   _____ c) face.

_____ b) palms.   _____ d) knees.

57. When the sebum hardens and the duct becomes clogged, a pore impaction called a(n) _____ is formed.

58. Name two functions of sebum.

1) _____

2) _____

59. List the principle functions of the skin.

a) _____

b) _____

c) _____

d) _____

e) _____

f) _____

60. Cosmetic products are formulated to penetrate the epidermis.

_____ True   _____ False

Promote Nutrition and Skin Health

61. Name the six classes of nutrients that the body needs.

1) _____

2) _____

3) _____

4) _____

5) _____

6) _____

62. The body makes all of the nutrients it needs.

_____ True   _____ False

63. The United States Department of Agriculture (USDA) developed a special program called MyPlate to help people determine the amounts of food they need to eat from the five basic food groups. What are the five basic food groups?

1) _____

2) _____

3) _____

4) _____

5) _____

64. To maintain a balanced diet, a person should eat a _____ of foods.

65. A healthy diet is high in _____, _____, and _____ products.

66. A healthy diet is low in _____, _____, and _____.

67. Prepared food products contain _____ and modified _____, which should be eaten in moderation.

68. A healthy diet should be balanced with the right amount of _____ _____.

69. Explain what information is found on a food label.

_____ _____ _____

_____

70. What does RDA stand for? _____

71. Vitamins are nutritional supplements, not cosmetic ingredients.

_____ True   _____ False

72. Some vitamins have been shown to have a positive effect on the skin's health when taken by mouth.

_____ True   _____ False

73. Match the following vitamin with its effect on healthy skin:

_____ 1. Vitamin A   a) Enables the body to properly absorb and use calcium, and promotes rapid healing of the skin

_____ 2. Vitamin C   b) Aids in the health, function, and repair of skin cells

_____ 3. Vitamin D   c) Helps protect the skin from the harmful effects of the sun's UV light

_____ 4. Vitamin E   d) Aids in and accelerates the skin's healing processes

74. The best way of making sure your body gets the nutrients it needs each day is to:

_____ a) take a nutritional supplement.   _____ c) avoid all fats.

_____ b) improve your diet.   _____ d) drink more water.

75. Water composes _____ of the body's weight.

76. The amount of water needed by an individual varies depending on:

a) _____

b) _____

77. Drinking pure water is essential to the health of the skin and body because it:

a) _____

b) _____

c) _____

d) _____

78. ⚕ **ACTIVITY:** Talk to your instructor and arrange a class competition based on you and your fellow students tracking your food and water intake over a period of one week. Keep a small, spiral note pad handy and write down everything you eat and drink throughout each day. Alternatively, you can download a free app on your cell phone that allows you to track your food and water intake. Be certain to note how much pure water you drink. When tracking your food intake, look at how many processed foods you eat compared to healthy foods, fruits, vegetables, and so on. While you may think you follow a fairly healthy diet at this time, logging your actual consumption may be an eye-opening event.

At the end of the week, the class will prepare a summary of their findings. In the space below, suggest new actions that you can take in order to be healthier. For example, making meals at home, having healthy snacks on hand, drinking more water than juices or soda, and so on. The instructor can grant awards to those who did the best, most complete job of tracking as well as having the healthiest food and water intake. Further, why not challenge your classmates to extend this revealing activity for a full month?

_____

_____

_____

_____

_____

_____

Date: _____

Rating: _____

Text Pages: 170–195

why study SKIN DISORDERS AND DISEASES?

1. Skin care specialists are in high demand in many salons and spas and earn excellent salaries.

   _____ True   _____ False

2. List the reasons a cosmetologist should study and have a thorough understanding of skin disorders and diseases.

   a) _____

   _____

   _____

   b) _____

   _____

   _____

   c) _____

   _____

   _____

Identify Disorders and Diseases of the Skin

3. A physician who specializes in diseases and disorders of the skin, hair, and nails is called a(n) _____.

4. A brand new client arrives at your salon for a facial, and you notice she has an inflamed red rash on her chin that she says is "nothing." What should you do?

_____ a) Perform a facial on the client as scheduled, going easy on the chin area

_____ b) Search online to see if you can identify whether the rash is contagious

_____ c) Tell her kindly that you cannot perform a facial without a note from her doctor permitting the service

5. Explain your answer to question 4.

_____

_____

_____

6. A mark on the skin that may indicate an injury or damage that changes the structure of tissues or organs is known as a(n) _____.

7. The two types of lesions are:

1) _____

2) _____

8. Match each of the following primary lesions with its description.

_____ 1. Bulla   a) Flat spot or discoloration on the skin

_____ 2. Cyst and Tubercle   b) Small blister or sac containing clear fluid, lying within or just beneath the epidermis

_____ 3. Macule   c) Abnormal mass varying in size, shape, and color

_____ 4. Nodule   d) Large blister containing a watery fluid

_____ 5. Papule   e) Itchy, swollen lesion that can be caused by a blow, scratch, insect bite, urticaria, or the sting of a nettle

_____ 6. Pustule   f) Raised, inflamed, papule with a white or yellow center containing pus

_____ 7. Tumor   h) Small elevation on the skin that contains no fluid

_____ 8. Vesicle   g) Closed, abnormally developed sac that contains pus, semifluid, or morbid matter, above or below the skin

_____ 9. Wheal   i) A solid bump larger than 0.4 inches (1 cm) that can be easily felt

9. A freckle is an example of a:

_____ a) bulla.   _____ c) papule.

_____ b) macule.   _____ d) tubercle.

10. Which of the following primary lesions requires a medical referral?

_____ a) Bulla   _____ c) Papule

_____ b) Macule   _____ d) Pustule

11. _____ lesions are characterized by piles of material on the skin surface or by depressions in the skin surface.

12. Match each of the following secondary lesions with its description.

_____ 1. Crust   a) Skin sore or abrasion produced by scratching or scraping

_____ 2. Excoriation   b) Thick scar resulting from excessive growth of fibrous tissue

_____ 3. Fissure   c) Slightly raised or depressed area on the skin that forms as a result of the healing process related to an injury or lesion

_____ 4. Keloid   d) Open lesion on the skin or mucous membrane of the body

_____ 5. Scale   e) Thin, dry, or oily plate of epidermal flakes

_____ 6. Scar   f) Crack in the skin that penetrates the dermis

_____ 7. Ulcer   g) Dead cells that form over a wound or blemish while it is healing

13. Identify the secondary skin lesions as illustrated:

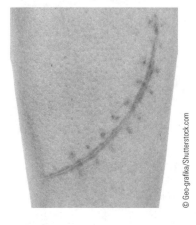

© Geo-grafika/Shutterstock.com

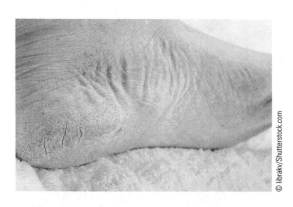

© librakv/Shutterstock.com

Clue: Slightly raised or depressed area of the skin that forms as a result of the healing process related to an injury or lesion.

Clue: Crack in the skin that penetrates the dermis.

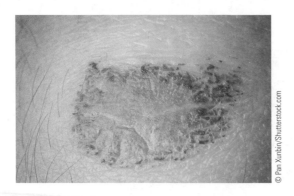

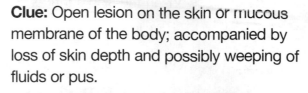

Clue: Dead cells that form over a wound or blemish while healing; accumulation of sebum and pus, sometimes mixed with epidermal cells.

Clue: Open lesion on the skin or mucous membrane of the body; accompanied by loss of skin depth and possibly weeping of fluids or pus.

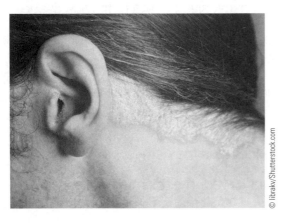

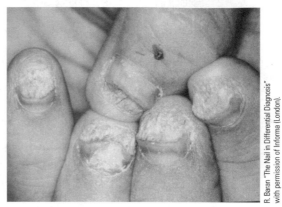

Clue: Thin, dry, or oily plate of epidermal flakes.

Clue: Skin sore or abrasion produced by scratching or scraping.

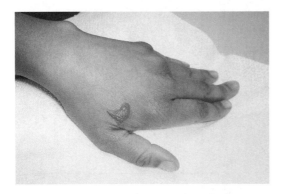

Clue: A thick scar resulting from excessive growth of fibrous tissue.

14. Give an example of a scale. _____

15. Where on the body are fissures most commonly found?

_____

16. Another term for scar is _____.

17. Which of the seven secondary lesions that were discussed in this chapter require medical referral? _____

Identify Disorders of the Sebaceous (Oil) Glands

18. An open comedo is also known as a _____.

19. Match each of the following disorders of the sebaceous glands with its description.

_____ 1. Comedo

_____ 2. Milia

_____ 3. Acne

_____ 4. Seborrheic dermatitis

_____ 5. Rosacea

_____ 6. Sebaceous cyst

a) Skin condition caused by an inflammation of the sebaceous glands

b) Chronic condition that appears primarily on the cheeks and nose

c) Hair follicle filled with keratin and sebum

d) Large, protruding pocket-like lesion filled with sebum

e) Chronic inflammation of the sebaceous glands caused by retained secretions and bacteria

f) Benign, keratin-filled cysts

20. Comedones can be removed by trained beauty professionals as long as proper procedures are employed and the procedure is performed in a clean environment.

_____ True   _____ False

21. Why does a whitehead not appear black?

_____

_____

_____

Identify Disorders of the Sudoriferous (Sweat) Glands

22. Match each of following disorders of the sudoriferous glands with its description.

_____ 1. Anhidrosis   a) Foul-smelling perspiration

_____ 2. Bromhidrosis   b) Excessive sweating

_____ 3. Hyperhidrosis   c) Deficiency in perspiration

_____ 4. Miliaria rubra   d) Prickly heat; acute inflammatory disorder of the sweat glands

Recognize Inflammations and Common Infections of the Skin

23. Match each of the following skin conditions with its description.

_____ 1. Dermatitis   a) Recurring viral infection that often presents as a fever blister or cold sore

_____ 2. Eczema   b) Inflammatory condition of the skin

_____ 3. Herpes simplex   c) Noncontagious skin disease characterized by red patches covered with silver-white scales

_____ 4. Psoriasis   d) Inflammatory, uncomfortable, and often chronic disease of the skin

_____ 5. Conjunctivitis   e) Contagious eye infection caused by bacteria or virus

_____ 6. Impetigo   f) Contagious bacterial skin infection characterized by weeping lesions

24. With treatment, the herpes simplex virus can be completely cured with all traces of the virus removed from the body.

_____ True   _____ False

25. It is possible to get eczema by working on a client who has this condition.

_____ True   _____ False

Recognize Pigment Disorders of the Skin

26. Name six factors that may affect the pigment of the skin.

    1) _____

    2) _____

    3) _____

    4) _____

    5) _____

    6) _____

27. What is the medical term for an abnormal coloration of the skin?

    _____

28. A darker than normal skin pigmentation appearing as dark splotches is called

    _____.

29. The absence of pigment resulting in light or white splotches on the skin is called

    _____.

30. Match each of the following skin pigmentation disorders with its description.

    _____ 1. Albinism   a) Hyperpigmentation on the skin in spots that are not elevated

    _____ 2. Chloasma   b) Small or large malformation of the skin due to abnormal pigmentation or dilated capillaries

    _____ 3. Lentigines   c) Absence of melanin pigment in the body

    _____ 4. Leukoderma   d) Abnormal brown- or wine-colored skin discoloration

    _____ 5. Nevus   e) Change in pigmentation caused by exposure to the sun or ultraviolet light

    _____ 6. Stain   f) Hereditary condition that causes milky white splotches of skin

    _____ 7. Tan   g) Skin disorder characterized by light, abnormal patches

    _____ 8. Vitiligo   h) Technical term for freckles

List Hypertrophies of the Skin

31. A _____ of the skin is an abnormal growth of the skin.

32. A skin growth that is _____ is harmless.

33. Match the each of the following skin abnormalities with its description.

_____ 1. Keratoma   a) A small brownish spot or blemish

_____ 2. Mole   b) A hypertrophy of the papillae and epidermis; a wart

_____ 3. Skin tag   c) A small brown- or flesh-colored outgrowth of the skin

_____ 4. Verruca   d) An acquired, superficial, thickened patch of epidermis

34. A more common name for a keratoma is _____; a keratoma that grows inward is called a(n) _____.

35. Who should remove a skin tag for a client? _____

36. Verruca can spread from one location to another, particularly along a scratch in the skin.

_____ True   _____ False

Understand Skin Cancer

37. Why has skin cancer become one of the most common causes of cancer-related deaths?

_____

_____

38. _____ is the most common type of skin cancer and is the least severe.

39. _____ is more serious and is often characterized by scaly red papules or nodules.

40. _____ is the most dangerous form of skin cancer and is often characterized by black or dark brown patches and may appear uneven in texture, jagged, or raised.

41. The least common form of skin cancer is _____.

42. Explain the role of the cosmetologist in detecting skin cancer.

_____

_____

_____

_____

_____

_____

43. List the parts of the ABCDE Cancer Checklist.

A: _____

B: _____

C: _____

D: _____

E: _____

Examine Acne and Problem Skin

44. Acne is considered both a skin _____ and a(n) _____ problem.

45. Acne may occur in a person of any age.

_____ True   _____ False

46. A predisposition to acne is based on:

a) _____

b) _____

47. People with acne inherit the tendency to retain cells that gather on the walls of the _____, eventually clumping and _____ the follicle.

48. What causes sebum to harden? _____

49. List four basic ways to treat minor forms of acne.

1) _____

_____

2) _____

_____

3) _____

_____

4) _____

_____

50. A product that is _____ has been designed and proven not to clog the follicles.

51. When is it appropriate for a salon professional to treat a mild or moderate case of acne?

_____

_____

_____

_____

Analyze Aging Skin Issues

52. Define intrinsic factors that influence skin aging and give three examples.

_____

_____

_____

_____

53. Describe extrinsic factors that influence skin aging and give six examples.

_____

_____

_____

_____

54. Explain why smoking and drinking, when done together, can be damaging to the skin.

_____

_____

_____

_____

55. Eating a well-balanced diet allows for all body systems to function at maximum performance and _____ the fragile tissues of the skin.

56. What is the best defense against pollutants affecting the skin?

_____

_____

_____

57. Damage done by lifestyle habits can be impossible to repair or diminish.

_____ True   _____ False

Understand the Sun and Its Effects

58. Approximately 80 to 85 percent of the symptoms of aging skin are caused by the accumulation of _____.

59. As we age, the _____ and _____ of the skin naturally weaken.

60. UV light is sometimes called a "UV ray" which is a shorter way of saying that it is a form of ___ _____ ____, and as such can be damaging.

61. UVA rays, also known as _____, are deep-penetrating rays that weaken the collagen and elastin fibers, causing _____ _____ of the tissues.

62. UVB rays, also known as _____, cause sunburns, tanning of the skin, and the majority of skin cancers.

63. List the precautions to take when you will be exposed to the sun.

a) _____

_____

b) _____

_____

c) _____

_____

d) _____

_____

e) _____

_____

f) _____

_____

Recognize Contact Dermatitis

64. A skin disorder that is the most common work-related skin disorder for all cosmetology professionals is _____.

65. Why are cosmetologists likely to have contact dermatitis?

_____

_____

_____

66. _____ is an allergic reaction created by repeated exposure to a chemical or a substance.

67. What must be done once an allergy to a product has been established?

_____

_____

_____

68. What are the three most likely places allergies may occur?

1) _____

2) _____

3) _____

69. If the epidermis is temporarily damaged by irritating substances, it is called

_____.

70. Name two types of products with irritant potential.

1) _____

2) _____

71. Explain what occurs when the skin is damaged by irritating substances.

_____

_____

_____

_____

_____

_____

72. Describe how cosmetologists can prevent both types of dermatitis while at work.

_____

_____

_____

_____

_____

_____

73. List at least three strategies cosmetologists should follow for self-protection and to avoid a skin problem.

1) _____

_____

2) _____

_____

3) _____

_____

4) _____

_____

74. **ACTIVITY:** Assemble a group of about five or six fellow students to conduct skin condition research. Using a magnifying glass, examine each other's skin for different types of skin conditions. Using a device such as a smart phone or digital camera, take photos of different conditions. Under each photo, list the technical term for the condition, what causes it, and what treatment can be used, if any, to treat it or state that it should be referred to a physician. Depending if you decide to print your photos or use them digitally, use your creativity to design a poster or PowerPoint slide show depicting "real-life" skin conditions.

_____

_____

_____

_____

_____

CHAPTER 9 NAIL STRUCTURE & GROWTH

Date: _____

Rating: _____

Text Pages: 196–205

why study NAIL STRUCTURE AND GROWTH?

1. List three reasons why cosmetologists should study and have a thorough understanding of nail structure and growth.

   1) _____

   _____

   2) _____

   _____

   3) _____

   _____

Distinguish the Structure of the Natural Nail

2. The _____ is the hard protective plate composed mainly of keratin, the fiber-shaped protein found in skin and hair, which is located at the end of the finger or toe.

3. Natural nails are appendages of the skin and part of the _____ system, which is made up of the skin and its various organs.

4. Nail plates protect the tips of the fingers and toes, and their appearance can reflect the _____ of the body.

5. Another name for the natural nail is the _____.

6. The natural nail is composed mainly of a protein called _____.

7. The keratin found in the natural nail is not as hard as the keratin found in the hair or skin.

_____ a) True   _____ b) False

8. Describe the appearance of a healthy nail. _____

_____

_____

_____

9. A healthy nail may look dry and hard, but its water content is actually between _____,
and varies according to the relative humidity of the surrounding environment.

_____ a) 5 and 10 percent   _____ c) 15 and 25 percent

_____ b) 10 and 20 percent   _____ d) 20 and 30 percent

10. The water content directly affects the nail's _____; the lower the water
content the more _____ the nail becomes.

11. What can be done to reduce water loss and improve flexibility?

_____

Identify Nail Anatomy

12. How many main parts is the natural nail unit divided into?

_____ a) Five   _____ b) Six   _____ c) Seven   _____ d) Nine

13. Together, all of the main parts of the nail are referred to as the _____

_____.

14. Identify the parts of the nail as illustrated below:

15. The nail plate is relatively _____ and will allow water to pass through it much more easily than through normal skin of an equal thickness.

16. The _____ is the most visible and functional part of the nail unit. It is constructed of about _____ layers of nail cells.

17. The part of the nail plate that extends over the tip of the finger or toe is the

_____.

18. Which of the following best describes the nail plate?

_____ a) Soft   _____ c) Dry

_____ b) Porous   _____ d) Dormant

19. The _____ is the portion of living skin that supports the nail plate as it grows toward the free edge.

20. The nail bed contains many nerves, and is attached to the nail plate by a thin layer of tissue called the _____.

21. The _____ is the area where the nail plate cells are formed.

22. The visible part of the matrix that extends from underneath the living skin is called the

_____.

23. Every nail has a lunula.

_____ True   _____ False

24. The whitish color of the lunula is caused by the _____ off the surface of the visible part of the underlying matrix.

25. Why is it sometimes difficult to see a lunula? _____

_____

26. Growth and appearance of the nails can be affected if any of the following conditions exist:

a) _____

b) _____

c) _____

27. The _____ is the dead, colorless tissue attached to the natural nail plate.

28. What is the purpose of the cuticle? _____

_____

_____

29. Which of the following best describes the cuticle?

_____ a) Alive   _____ c) Difficult to remove

_____ b) Pigmented   _____ d) Unimportant

30. Which of the following is most likely to need a softener?

_____ a) Cuticle   _____ b) Eponychium

31. The living skin at the base of the natural nail plate covering the matrix area is the

_____.

32. Describe the difference between the eponychium and the cuticle.

_____

_____

33. The cuticle will bleed if it is cut.

_____ True   _____ False

34. Which of the following can be removed with gentle scraping?

_____ a) Cuticle   _____ b) Eponychium

35. The _____ is the slightly thickened layer of skin under the nail that lies between the fingertip and the free edge of the nail plate.

36. What is the function of the hyponychium?   _____

_____

_____

37. A tough band of fibrous tissue that connects bones or holds an organ in place is called a _____.

38. Specialized ligaments attach the nail bed and _____ to the underlying bone and are located at the base of the matrix and around the edges of the nail bed.

39. The _____ are folds of normal skin that surround the nail plate and which form nail grooves.

40. What are nail grooves? _____

41. The fold of skin that overlaps the side of the nail is called the _____.

Discuss Nail Growth

42. The growth and health of the nail plate is affected by _____

    _____.

43. Describe services a cosmetologist may perform to help make a client's nail plate thicker. _____

    _____

    _____

    _____

44. Explain why toenails are thicker than fingernails. _____

    _____

45. Identify the various shapes of nails in the illustration below:

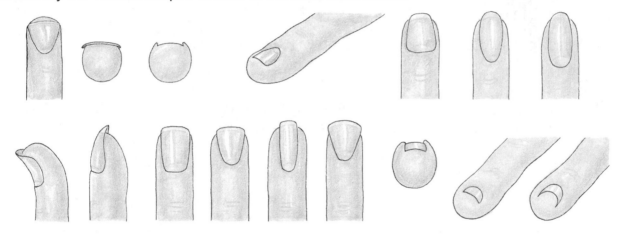

46. The average rate of nail plate growth in the normal adult is about:

    _____ a) $\frac{1}{4}$ to $\frac{1}{2}$ inch per month.   _____ c) $\frac{1}{10}$ to $\frac{1}{8}$ inch per month.

    _____ b) $\frac{1}{2}$ to $\frac{3}{4}$ inch per week.   _____ d) $\frac{1}{8}$ to $\frac{1}{6}$ inch per week.

47. Nails grow faster in the winter than they do in the summer.

    _____ True   _____ False

48. Compared with the nails of an average adult, children's nails grow more rapidly, while elderly adults' nails grow at a slower rate.

    _____ True   _____ False

49. The nail of the middle finger grows fastest and the thumbnail grows the slowest.

    _____ True   _____ False

50. What causes the growth rates of the nail to increase dramatically during pregnancy?

_____

51. A pregnant woman who is taking prenatal vitamins will experience even more rapid nail growth than a pregnant women who is not taking prenatal vitamins.

_____ True   _____ False

52. What will cause an abnormal shape or form of the nail?

_____

_____

53. How long does replacement of the natural fingernail take?

_____

_____

54. Toenails take _____ months to be fully replaced.

_____ a) three to five   _____ c) seven to nine

_____ b) five to seven   _____ d) nine to twelve

55. Like hair, the nail will automatically shed periodically.

_____ True   _____ False

Know Your Nails

56. A licensed cosmetologist is allowed to:

_____ treat nail disorders.

_____ remove ingrown toenails.

_____ work on healthy nails only.

57. The act of typing on a keyboard or lightly touching natural nails on piano keys stimulates the nails and makes them grow. Why do you think this is the case? Once you have considered your answer, find out if you are correct by conducting an Internet search on the topic.

_____

_____

_____

_____

_____

_____

58. **ACTIVITY:** After unscrambling the terms listed below, match them up with the appropriate description or clue.

Scrambled Terms:		Clue Number
latutan anli: _____		_____
citucel: _____		_____
aximrt: _____		_____
auunll: _____		_____
ichmuyeonp: _____		_____
ichmuyhpon: _____		_____
repnoiycmiuh: _____		_____
eerf gdee: _____		_____
magilten: _____		_____
deb muilpithee: _____		_____

Clues:

1) Tough fibrous tissue that connects bones

2) Visible part of the matrix extending from underneath the living skin

3) Dead, colorless tissue attached to the natural nail plate

4) The living tissue bordering the root and sides of a fingernail or toenail

5) Guides the nail plate along the nail bed as it grows

6) Also known as onyx

7) Living skin at the base of the natural nail plate that covers the matrix area

8) Part of the nail plate that extends over the tip of the finger or toe

9) Slightly thickened layer of skin under the nail between the fingertip and free edge

10) Area where the nail plate cells are formed

CHAPTER 10

NAIL DISORDERS & DISEASES

Date: _____

Rating: _____

Text Pages: 206–221

1 Nails may be described as small _____ into an individual's general health.

2. Certain health conditions may first be revealed by a change in the nails, a visible disorder, or poor nail growth.

_____ True   _____ False

3. Some conditions are easily treated in the salon such as ingrown toenails.

_____ True   _____ False

why study NAIL DISORDERS AND DISEASES?

4. List the reasons why a cosmetologist should study and have a thorough understanding of nail disorders and diseases.

a) _____

_____

_____

b) _____

_____

_____

c) _____

_____

_____

Pinpoint Common and Uncommon Nail Disorders

5. Describe a normal healthy nail. _____

_____

_____

_____

6. A _____ is a condition caused by injury, heredity, or previous disease of the nail unit.

7. You can help your clients with nail disorders in what two ways?

1) _____

_____

2) _____

_____

8. When should a client with a nail disorder not receive services? _____

_____ What should you do if any of these are

present? _____

_____

9. Visible depressions running across the width of the natural nail plate are
_____. They usually result from _____ or
_____ that has traumatized the body.

10. _____ are a condition in which a blood clot forms under the nail plate, causing a dark purplish spot.

11. List at least three possible causes of discolored nails.

1) _____

2) _____

3) _____

4) _____

12. A noticeably thin, white nail plate that is much more flexible than normal is known as
a(n) _____; this condition is usually caused by _____

_____.

13. Describe the process of manicuring an eggshell nail. _____

_____

_____

_____

_____

14. A(n) _____ is a condition in which the living skin around the nail plate splits and tears.

15. What will aid in correcting hangnails? _____ _____

_____

_____

16. Under what circumstances should a cosmetologist intentionally cut or tear a client's living skin?

_____ a) Only when requested to by the client

_____ b) Only if the client has an infected hangnail

_____ c) Whenever the skin appears to be dry or rough looking

_____ d) Under no circumstances

17. Name four signs of infection.

1) _____

2) _____

3) _____

4) _____

18. Koilonychia are hard spoon nails with a concave shape that appear scooped out.

_____ True _____ False

19. White spots, or _____ spots, are whitish discolorations of the nails, usually caused by minor injury to the nail matrix.

20. The darkening of the fingernails or toenails is _____.

21. _____, or bitten nails, is the result of a person's habit of chewing the nail or the hardened, damaged skin surrounding the nail plate.

22. The condition of split or brittle nails that have a series of lengthwise ridges giving a rough appearance to the surface of the nail plate is _____.

23. Onychorrhexis is usually caused by:

a) _____

b) _____

c) _____

d) _____

e) _____

24. It is never appropriate to apply a nail enhancement product if a client's nail bed is exposed.

_____ True   _____ False

25. Plicatured nail, also known as _____, is a type of highly curved nail plate usually caused by injury to the _____, but it may be

_____.

26. _____ are vertical lines running down the length of the natural nail plate that are caused by _____ of the nails, usually the result of

_____.

27. What can be done to minimize the appearance of ridges?

a) _____

b) _____

28. Splinter hemorrhages are caused by physical trauma or injury to the

_____.

29. Explain why splinter hemorrhages are always positioned lengthwise in the direction of

nail growth. _____

_____

_____

30. An abnormal condition that occurs when the skin is stretched by the nail plate is

_____.

31. The terms *cuticle* and *pterygium* are the same thing and may be used interchangeably.

_____ True   _____ False

32. Nail pterygium is caused by damage to the _____

or _____ and should not be treated by pushing the

extension of skin back with an instrument.

33. Explain the proper way to care for nail pterygium. _____

_____

34. Nail plates with a deep or sharp curvature at the free edge have this shape because of the _____; this is known as a _____.

Recognize Nail Diseases

35. Match each of the following nail diseases with its description.

_____ 1. Onychosis

a) Ingrown nails

_____ 2. Onychia

b) The separation and falling off of a nail plate from the nail bed

_____ 3. Onychocryptosis

c) A bacterial inflammation of the tissues surrounding the nail

_____ 4. Onycholysis

d) A red, itchy rash on the skin on the bottoms of the feet and/or between the toes

_____ 5. Onychomadesis

e) A severe inflammation of the nail in which a lump of red tissue grows up from the nail bed to the nail plate

_____ 6. Nail psoriasis

f) Any deformity or disease of the natural nail

_____ 7. Paronychia

g) The lifting of the nail plate from the nail bed without shedding

_____ 8. Pyogenic granuloma

h) A fungal infection of the natural nail plate

_____ 9. Tinea pedis

i) Tiny pits or severe roughness on the surface of the nail plate

_____ 10. Onychomycosis

j) An inflammation of the nail matrix followed by shedding of the nail

36. Are there any nail diseases that should be treated in the salon?

_____ Yes   _____ No

37. People who work in jobs that require them to regularly place their hands in _____ are more likely to develop nail infections.

38. _____ are parasites that, under some circumstances, may cause infections of the feet and hands.

39. Why is nail fungi of concern to a salon? _____

_____

40. Which of the following statements is most accurate?

_____ a) It is highly likely that a client with a nail fungus could infect a cosmetologist

_____ b) Fungal infections of the fingernail are more common than fungal infections of the toenail

_____ c) A client with a fungal infection of the toenail could potentially infect another client

41. Fungal infections prefer to grow in conditions where the skin is warm, dry, and dark, that is, on feet inside shoes.

_____ True   _____ False

42. How can the transmission of fungal infections be avoided? _____

_____

43. A bartender is most likely to develop which of the following nail infections?

_____ a) Onychomadesis   _____ c) Onycholysis

_____ b) Paronychia   _____ d) Onychocryptosis

44. The green, yellow, or black discoloration on a nail bed is usually a(n) _____ infection.

45. In the past, discolorations of the nail plate were incorrectly referred to as

_____.

46. Describe the stages of a typical bacterial infection of the nail plate.

_____

_____

47. When is it appropriate for a cosmetologist to treat a client's nail infection?

_____ a) Only if asked by the salon manager

_____ b) Under no circumstances

_____ c) If the client is unable to see a physician

_____ d) In cases where the infection appears mild

48. Bacterial infections under nail enhancements are a result of moisture trapped between the natural nail and the nail enhancements.

_____ True   _____ False

49. Which of the following conditions is usually caused by trauma, physical injury, or allergic reaction of the nail bed?

_____ a) Nail psoriasis   _____ c) Onycholysis

_____ b) Paronychia   _____ d) Onychomycosis

Perform Hand, Nail, and Skin Analysis

50. Performing a hand and nail analysis on a client is only important on the first visit to the salon.

_____ True   _____ False

51. What is the first step in performing a hand, nail, and skin analysis?

_____ a) Observe the temperature of the skin.

_____ b) Observe the moisture level of the skin.

_____ c) Clean the hands of both the cosmetologist and the client.

_____ d) Determine if the client has any pain.

52. ACTIVITY: Play the "Who Am I?" game. Use colored construction paper or card stock and a large marker and write the terms of each of the nail disorders and diseases learned in this chapter on one side and the definition of the term on the opposite side. Enlist your fellow students in the activity to learn all the terms. Using a straight pin or safety pin, attach one term to the back of each student without telling that student what the term is. Throughout the day, other students should provide small clues to the student about the term until he or she is able to determine who he or she is (what the term is). Be creative in how you provide clues and make it fun.

_____

_____

_____

_____

CHAPTER 11

PROPERTIES OF THE HAIR & SCALP

Date: _____

Rating: _____

Text Pages: 222–251

why study PROPERTIES OF THE HAIR AND SCALP?

1. All professional hair services must be based on a thorough understanding of the growth, _____, and composition of hair.

2. List below why it is important for a cosmetologist to study and understand the properties of the hair and scalp.

   a) _____

   _____

   _____

   b) _____

   _____

   _____

   c) _____

   _____

   _____

Discover the Structure of Hair

3. _____ is the scientific study of hair and its diseases and care, which comes from the Greek words _____, meaning "hair," and _____, meaning "the study of."

4. A mature strand of human hair is divided into two parts: the _____, located below the surface of the epidermis, and the _____, the portion of the hair that projects above the epidermis.

5. Match the five main structures of the hair root with their description.

_____ 1. Hair follicle

_____ 2. Hair bulb

_____ 3. Dermal papilla

_____ 4. Arrector pili muscle

_____ 5. Sebaceous glands

a) Small, cone-shaped elevation located at the base of the hair follicle that fits into the hair bulb

b) The tube-like depression or pocket in the skin or scalp that contains the hair root

c) Small, involuntary muscle in the base of the hair follicle

d) The oil glands in the skin that are connected to the hair follicles

e) The thickened, club-shaped structure that forms the lower part of the root

6. Hair follicles are distributed all over the body, with the exceptions of:

a) _____

b) _____

7. More than one hair will never grow from a single follicle.

_____ True   _____ False

8. The lowest part of the hair strand is called the hair _____.

9. Which part of the hair root contains the blood and nerve supply that provides the nutrients needed for hair growth? _____

10. Which muscle causes goose bumps when it contracts due to strong emotions or a cold sensation? _____

11. The sebaceous glands secrete a fatty or an oily substance called _____, which lubricates the skin.

12. Identify the parts of the skin and hair illustrated below:

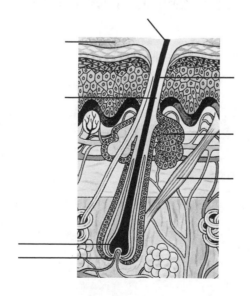

13. What are the three main layers of the hair shaft?

    1) _____

    2) _____

    3) _____

14. Identify the cross-sections of the hair cuticle as illustrated below:

15. The outermost layer of the hair is the _____.

16. Describe the hair cuticle layer. _____

    _____

    _____

17. Describe what a healthy cuticle layer protects. _____

    _____

    _____

18. If you hold the end of a single strand of hair in one hand and then grasp it between the thumb and forefinger of the other hand and move them down the hair shaft, the hair will feel _____.

19. Why must oxidation haircolors, permanent waving solutions, and chemical hair relaxers have an alkaline pH? _____

    _____

    _____

20. Which layer of the hair is the cortex? _____

21. What percentage of the total weight of hair comes from the cortex?

    _____ a) 50 percent   _____ c) 80 percent

    _____ b) 70 percent   _____ d) 90 percent

22. Name three different hair properties for which the cortex is responsible.

1) _____

2) _____

3) _____

23. In what layer of the hair do changes involving oxidation haircoloring, wet setting, thermal styling, permanent waving, and chemical hair relaxing take place?

_____

24. The _____ is the innermost layer of the hair and is composed of round cells.

25. All hair has three layers of the hair shaft.

_____ True   _____ False

26. All male beard hair contains a medulla.

_____ True   _____ False

27. The medulla is involved in salon services.

_____ True   _____ False

Learn About the Chemical Composition of Hair

28. Hair is composed of _____ that grows from cells originating within the hair follicle.

29. The maturation of these cells is a process called _____.

30. Hair is a living thing.

_____ True   _____ False

Explain your answer:

_____

_____

_____

31. List the main elements that make up human hair and their percentage in normal hair.

a) _____

b) _____

c) _____

d) _____

e) _____

32. Together, the five elements that make up human hair are referred to as the
_____ elements to help people remember them; they are also found in
the _____ and the _____.

33. Match each of the following terms with its description.

_____ 1. Amino acids   a) The strong, chemical bond that joins amino acids

_____ 2. Helix   b) Units that are joined together and make up proteins

_____ 3. Peptide bond   c) A long chain of amino acids linked by peptide
bonds

_____ 4. Polypeptide chain   d) The spiral shape of a coiled protein

34. Polypeptide chains are cross-linked like the rungs on a ladder by three different types of
side bonds called:

1) _____

2) _____

3) _____

35. A _____ bond is a weak, physical, cross-link side
bond that is easily broken by water or heat; these bonds reform when the hair
_____.

36. Weak, physical, cross-linked side bonds between adjacent polypeptide chains are
_____ bonds.

37. A _____ bond is a strong, chemical side bond that joins the sulfur atoms
of two neighboring cysteine amino acids to create one cystine.

38. How are the hair's strong chemical side bonds broken?

_____

_____

_____

39. _____ are the tiny grains of pigment in the cortex that give natural color
to the hair. List and describe the two different types.

1) _____

2) _____

_____

40. How is gray hair different from other hair colors?

_____

_____

_____

41. The _____ of hair refers to the shape of the hair strand and is described as _____, _____, _____, or _____.

42. Natural wave patterns are the result of _____.

43. Asians and Native Americans tend to have extremely _____ hair, while African Americans tend to have _____ hair; however, anyone of any race, or mixed race, can have hair with varying degrees of curl.

44. In extremely curly hair, cross-sections appear _____ and vary in shape and thickness along their length.

45. The shape of a cross-section of hair always relates to the amount of curl in the hair.

_____ True _____ False

46. Extremely curly hair often has _____ elasticity.

The Truth About Hair Growth

47. The two main types of hair found on the body are _____ hair and _____ hair.

48. Describe vellus hair. _____

_____

49. On adults, vellus hair is usually found on the _____

_____

_____.

50. Men retain _____ vellus hair than women.

51. Describe terminal hair. _____

_____

52. Terminal hair is found on the _____.

53. All hair follicles are capable of producing either vellus or terminal hair, depending on genetics, age, and hormones.

_____ True   _____ False

54. Unscramble these words, and then match each word with its correct description.

gloeten   neanag   agatecn

_____ The growth phase of new hair

_____ The transition period between the growth and resting phases

_____ The resting phase

55. What is the average growth of healthy scalp hair per month?

_____ a) ¼ inch (0.6 cm)   _____ c) ¾ inch (1.8 cm)

_____ b) ½ inch (1.25 cm)   _____ d) 1 inch (2.5 cm)

56. When does scalp hair tend to grow most rapidly?

_____ a) Between the ages of 8 and 13

_____ b) Between the ages of 15 and 20

_____ c) Between the ages of 15 and 30

_____ d) Between the ages of 40 and 50

57. What percentage of scalp hair is in the catagen phase at any one time?

_____ a) Less than 1 percent   _____ c) 10 percent

_____ b) 5 percent   _____ d) 15 percent

58. What percentage of scalp hair is in the telogen phase at any one time?

_____ a) Less than 1 percent   _____ c) A little less than 10 percent

_____ b) 4 to 5 percent   _____ d) More than 15 percent

59. How long does the anagen phase generally last?

_____

60. Shaving, clipping, and cutting the hair makes it grow back faster, darker, and coarser.

_____ True   _____ False

61. Scalp massage increases hair growth.

_____ True   _____ False

62. Gray hair is coarser and more resistant than pigmented hair.

_____ True   _____ False

63. A cross-section of hair can be almost any shape, and its shape does not necessarily relate to the amount of curl or the shape of the follicle.

_____ True   _____ False

Understand Hair Loss Causes and Treatments

64. Under normal circumstances, everyone loses some hair every day.

_____ True   _____ False

65. According to recent measurements, the average rate of hair loss is _____ hairs per day.

66. Describe how bald and balding men are perceived by others.

_____

_____

_____

67. Abnormal hair loss is not as common in women as in men, but it can be very traumatic and devastating for women who experience it.

_____ True   _____ False

68. Abnormal hair loss is called _____.

69. _____ is the result of genetics, age, or hormonal changes that cause terminal hair to _____.

70. In men, androgenic alopecia is known as _____ and usually progresses to the familiar horseshoe-shaped fringe of hair.

71. By the age of 35, 40 percent of men and women show some degree of _____.

72. How many people does androgenic alopecia affect in the United States?

_____ a) Millions   _____ b) Thousands   _____ c) Hundreds

73. What is alopecia areata? _____

_____

_____

74. Alopecia areata that progresses to total scalp hair loss it is called _____ _____. When it results in complete body hair loss, it is called _____.

75. Jane, a client at your salon, gave birth to her first baby three months ago. When she comes in for a service, she complains that her hair seems to be shedding. This condition is called _____. You reassure Jane that her hair growth cycle should eventually return to _____ within about _____ after the baby is delivered.

76. What are the only two products that have been proven to stimulate hair growth and are approved by the Food and Drug Administration (FDA) for sale in the United States?

_____

77. A topical medication that is put on the scalp twice a day, and is sold over the counter as a nonprescription drug, is _____; the most commonly known product that contains this drug is called Rogaine®.

78. _____ is an oral prescription medication for men only and is more effective and convenient than its nonprescription counterpart.

79. Why are pregnant women warned against having any contact with the oral prescription medication used to treat hair loss in men?

_____

_____

_____

80. Describe the most common permanent treatment for hair loss.

_____

_____

_____

81. What nonmedical options can a hairstylist offer to counter hair loss?

_____

82. Summarize the different possible causes of hair loss.

_____

_____

_____

_____

Recognize Disorders of the Hair

83. Match each of the following hair disorders with its description.

_____ 1. Canities   a) A condition of abnormal growth of hair

_____ 2. Ringed hair   b) Technical term for gray hair

_____ 3. Hypertrichosis   c) Technical term for knotted hair

_____ 4. Trichoptilosis   d) Technical term for beaded hair

_____ 5. Trichorrhexis nodosa   e) Technical term for brittle hair

_____ 6. Monilethrix   f) Characterized by alternating bands of gray and pigmented hair

_____ 7. Fragilitas crinium   g) Technical term for split ends

84. There are two types of canities. They are _____ canities and _____ canities.

85. In addition to genetics, _____ and _____ may also cause premature gray hair.

86. What is an example of hypertrichosis? _____ What are possible treatments? _____

_____

_____

87. Softening the hair with conditioners and moisturizers is often used in the treatment of _____ and may also help _____, but will not repair split ends.

88. Abnormal hair loss may also be a side effect of _____ or _____ cancer treatments.

Recognize Disorders of the Scalp

89. How many pounds of dead skin does the average person shed each year?

_____

90. What is the difference between dry scalp and dandruff?

_____

_____

91. Name some causes of dry scalp. _____

_____

_____

92. Research confirms that dandruff is the result of a fungus called _____,
a naturally occurring fungus that is present on all human skin.

93. What can be done to control dandruff? _____

_____

94. List the two principle types of dandruff and give their characterizations.

1) _____

_____

2) _____

_____

95. What is seborrheic dermatitis? _____

_____

96. It is appropriate for a cosmetologist to perform a service on a client who has a severe
case of dandruff.

_____ True   _____ False

97. What does tinea look like? _____

_____

98. Tinea is contagious.

_____ True   _____ False

99. Ringworm is caused by a parasite.

_____ True   _____ False

100. What does tinea barbae affect? _____

_____

101. Which of the following conditions has a distinctive odor?

_____ a) Tinea barbae   _____ c) Scutula

_____ b) Scabies   _____ d) Head lice

102. List the ways head lice are transmitted from an infected person to a noninfected person. _____

_____

_____

103. As a cosmetologist, what are two ways you can help prevent the spread of infectious conditions? _____

_____

_____

_____

104. Match each of the following scalp disorders with its definition.

_____ 1. Pityriasis   a) Technical term for ringworm

_____ 2. Tinea   b) Dry, sulfur-yellow, cuplike crusts on the scalp called scutula

_____ 3. Tinea capitis   c) An acute, localized bacterial infection of the hair follicle

_____ 4. Tinea favosa   d) Technical term for dandruff

_____ 5. Scabies   e) An inflammation of the subcutaneous tissue caused by staphylococci

_____ 6. Pediculosis capitis   f) Fungal infection characterized by red papules, or spots, at the opening of the hair follicles

_____ 7. Furuncle   g) The infestation of the hair and scalp with head lice

_____ 8. Carbuncle   h) Caused by a parasite called a mite

Learn How to Perform a Thorough Hair and Scalp Analysis

105. What special tools does a cosmetologist need in order to perform a hair analysis?

_____

_____

106. List and define the four most important factors to consider in hair analysis.

1) _____

_____

2) _____

_____

3) _____

_____

4) _____

_____

107. What are the classifications of hair texture?

a) _____

b) _____

c) _____

108. All hair on a person's head has the same texture.

_____ True   _____ False

109. Which hair texture has the largest diameter? _____

110. Which hair texture is the most common and is the standard to which other hair is compared to?   _____

111. Which hair texture has the smallest diameter and is more fragile?

_____

112. Which hair texture usually requires extra processing when applying a product like haircolor? _____

113. Hair density can be classified as:

a) _____

b) _____

c) _____

114. Hair density and hair texture are essentially the same thing.

_____ True   _____ False

115. The average hair density is about _____ hairs per one square inch, and the average head of hair contains about _____ individual hair strands.

116. Which hair color typically has the lowest density?

_____ a) Brown   _____ c) Red

_____ b) Blond   _____ d) Black

117. The hair's ability to absorb moisture is its _____.

118. The degree of porosity is directly related to _____.

     Why? _____

     _____

     _____

119. A term that means resistant to being penetrated by moisture is _____;
     a term that means easily absorbs moisture is _____.

120. Hair with average porosity is considered _____. Overly porous hair is

     _____.

121. Chemical services performed on overly porous hair require _____

     _____.

122. Hair texture always indicates the hair's porosity; for example, coarse hair always has a
     low porosity.

     _____ True   _____ False

123. Describe how to check porosity. _____

     _____

     _____

     _____

124. In a porosity check, if the hair feels smooth, the cuticle is _____

     _____.

125. In a porosity check, if you can feel a slight roughness, the hair is considered

     _____.

126. In a porosity check, if the hair feels very rough, dry or breaks, it is considered

     _____.

127. The ability of the hair to stretch and return to its original length without breaking is its

     _____.

128. Hair elasticity is an indication of _____

     _____.

129. Wet hair with normal elasticity will stretch up to _____ of its original
     length and return without breaking. Dry hair stretches about _____ of
     its length.

130. Which of the following statements is true of hair with low elasticity?

_____ a) Chemical services will require a solution with a higher pH

_____ b) Hair services should not be performed at all

_____ c) It may not hold a permanent wave as easily

131. Hair growth patterns are caused by follicles that grow perpendicular (90-degree angle) to the scalp.

_____ True _____ False

132. During the hair analysis, the cosmetologist should identify any and all hair growth patterns and take them into consideration when creating the overall look, haircut, or hairstyle the client wants to achieve.

_____ True _____ False

133. Match each of the following terms with its description.

_____ 1) Hair stream   a. Hair flowing in the same direction

_____ 2) Whorl   b. Due to a particular pattern on hair stream on the forehead

_____ 3) Cowlick   c. Hair stream that spirals outward from a central point.

134. Which of the following is not a cause of dry hair and scalp?

_____ a) Excessive shampooing   _____ c) Inactive sebaceous glands

_____ b) Dry climate   _____ d) Active sebaceous glands

135. Dry hair and scalp can be caused by inactive _____ and is aggravated by excessive _____.

136. Oily hair and scalp is caused by _____ or _____ sebaceous glands.

137. Oily hair and scalp is characterized by _____

_____.

138. (W) **ACTIVITY:** Using the chart on page 127, perform a scalp and hair analysis on yourself and several other individuals such as other students, friends, or family members. Evaluate each scalp for conditions such as oiliness and shine, fullness, tightness, flakes or dryness and so forth. Analyze the hair density (thin, medium, thick/dense). Record any applicable disorders (e.g., canities, ringed hair, trichoptilosis, monilethrix, and so on) Part the hair from the center front of the forehead to the nape and then from the top of the ear over the apex to the top of the other ear. Take two or three hairs from each section of hair to evaluate the texture (fine, medium, coarse), the porosity (low, average, high), and the elasticity (low, normal, high). Based on your findings, record your treatment recommendations (shampoo type, conditioning treatments, and so on) for each individual.

Note: The second column in the chart has been filled out as an example only.

NAME	Jane Doe			
Scalp Analysis	Dry and scaly			
Hair Density	Medium			
Disorders of the Hair (if applicable)	Trichoptilosis			
Front Left: **Texture** **Porosity** **Elasticity**	Fine Low Low			
Back Left: **Texture** **Porosity** **Elasticity**	Fine Average Normal			
Front Right **Texture** **Porosity** **Elasticity**	Fine Low Low			
Back Right **Texture** **Porosity** **Elasticity**	Fine Average Normal			
Treatment	Avoid frequent shampooing and strong soaps; use moisturizing conditioning treatments			

Date: _____

Rating: _____

Text Pages: 252–271

why study CHEMISTRY?

1. When you first began studying to become a cosmetologist were you surprised that you would be learning about chemistry? Describe your reaction and why you think it is important for you to learn the basics about chemistry.

   _____

   _____

   _____

   _____

2. List three important reasons for studying and understanding chemistry as a cosmetologist.

   1) _____

   _____

   2) _____

   _____

   3) _____

   _____

Recognize How the Science of Chemistry Influences Cosmetology

3. _____ is the science that deals with the composition, structures, and properties of matter and how matter changes under different conditions.

4. _____ is the study of substances that contain the element carbon.

5. The term organic does not mean "natural."

_____ True   _____ False

6. Anything that is called *organic* is healthy and safe.

_____ True   _____ False

7. _____ is the study of substances that do not contain the element carbon but may contain the element hydrogen.

8. For each of the following substances, write an *O* if the item is organic and write an *I* if the item is inorganic.

_____ Gasoline   _____ Iron

_____ Water   _____ Air

_____ Synthetic fabrics   _____ Pesticides

_____ Shampoo

9. Explain why most inorganic substances do not burn, yet organic substances will burn. _____

_____

_____

Define Matter

10. Match each of the following terms with its definition.

_____ 1. Matter   a) Simplest form of chemical matter

_____ 2. Element   b) Chemical combination of two or more atoms

_____ 3. Atom   c) Any substance that occupies space and has mass

_____ 4. Molecule   d) The basic unit of matter

11. All matter has physical and chemical properties and exists in the form of a(n) _____, _____, or _____.

12. Everything that is made out of matter is:

_____ a) organic.   _____ b) a chemical.   _____ c) inorganic.

13. _____ does not occupy space or have mass.

14. Everything that is known to exist in the universe is made of either _____ or _____.

15. There are 118 known elements today and of these _____ occur naturally and the rest are produced by synthetic methods from nuclear reactions.

16. How are elements identified? _____ List the symbol for the following elements.

_____ Oxygen _____ Carbon _____ Hydrogen _____ Nitrogen _____ Sulfur

17. A(n) _____ is the smallest chemical component of an element and are structures that make up the element and have the same properties of that element.

18. Atoms cannot be divided into simpler substances by ordinary _____ means.

19. How are molecules made? _____

20. _____ contain two or more atoms of the same element in definite proportions.

21. _____ are a chemical combination of two or more atoms of different elements in definite proportions.

22. The nucleus of an atom consists of protons and neutrons and the number of protons determines the element.

_____ True _____ False

23. _____ are the three different physical forms of matter.

24. Match the three different states of matter with their corresponding characteristics.

_____ 1. Solids   a) Have no volume or shape

_____ 2. Liquids   b) Have a fixed shape and volume

_____ 3. Gases   c) Have a definite volume but take the shape of its container

25. What is an example of a(n) _____ that can exist in all _____ forms of matter. _____

_____.

26. _____ are characteristics that can be determined without a chemical reaction and do not involve a chemical change in the substance. Physical properties include _____

_____.

27. _____ are characteristics that can only be determined by a chemical reaction and a chemical change in the substance.

28. List at least two examples of chemical properties.

    1) _____

    _____

    2) _____

    _____

    3) _____

    _____

29. A change in the form or physical properties of a substance, without a chemical reaction or the creation of a new substance, is a(n) _____.

30. What are two examples of a physical change?

    1) _____

    2) _____

31. A change in the chemical composition or make-up of a substance is a(n) _____.

32. What is oxidation? _____

_____

33. List two examples of a chemical change.

    1) _____

    _____

    2) _____

    _____

34. *Redox* stands for _____ reaction.

35. Explain what happens during redox. _____

_____

36. What is an example of an oxidizing agent? _____

37. What is an example of a reducing agent? _____

_____

_____

_____

_____

38. Define each of the following terms.

a) Oxidizing agent _____

_____

b) Reducing agent _____

_____

c) Oxidation-reduction _____

_____

39. Redox reactions are responsible for the chemical changes created by haircolors, hair lighteners, permanent wave solutions, and thioglycolic acid neutralizers.

_____ True _____ False

40. Chemical reactions that release a significant amount of heat are called _____

_____.

41. All oxidation reactions are exothermic reactions.

_____ True _____ False

42. _____ is the rapid oxidation of a substance accompanied by the production of heat and light.

43. A _____ is a chemical combination of matter in definite proportions.

44. Give an example of a pure substance. _____

_____

45. A physical mixture is a physical combination of _____ in any proportion.

46. Salt water is an example of a:

_____ a) pure substance. _____ b) physical mixture.

47. Describe three ways a physical mixture is different from a pure substance.

_____

_____

_____

48. Match each of the following terms with its description.

_____ 1. Solution   a) Stable physical mixture of two or more substances in a solvent

_____ 2. Solute   b) The substance that dissolves the solute and makes the solution

_____ 3. Solvent   c) The substance that is dissolved into a solution

49. Which of the following is known as the universal solvent?

_____ a) Water   _____ b) Oil   _____ c) Alcohol

50. _____ liquids are mutually soluble, meaning that they can be mixed together to form clear solutions.

51. _____ liquids are not capable of being mixed together to form stable solutions.

52. Determine whether the following combinations of liquid are miscible (*M*) liquid, or immiscible (*I*).

_____ a) Water and alcohol   _____ b) Water and oil   _____ c) Water and salt

53. An unstable physical mixture of undissolved particles in a liquid is:

_____ a) an emulsion.   _____ b) a suspension.   _____ c) a surfactant.

54. An unstable physical mixture of two or more immiscible substances plus an emulsifier is:

_____ a) an emulsion.   _____ b) a suspension.   _____ c) a surfactant.

55. Substances that allow oil and water to mix or emulsify are:

_____ a) emulsions.   _____ b) suspensions.   _____ c) surfactants.

56. Give two examples of a suspension.

1) _____

2) _____

57. Which of the following is true about an emulsion?

_____ a) It never separates   _____ c) Nail primer is an example

_____ b) It is stable   _____ d) It separates very slowly

58. A surfactant molecule has two distinct parts. The head is _____, meaning water-loving, and the tail is _____, meaning oil-loving.

59. What does the term *surfactant* stand for? _____

60. What is the common characteristic of solutions and suspensions?

_____

61. Powdered hair lighteners are physical mixtures that may _____ during shipping and storage and should be thoroughly mixed by shaking the container before each use.

62. What are two examples of a water-in-oil emulsion? _____

_____

63. Give four examples of semisolid physical mixtures that may be used in the salon.

1) _____

2) _____

3) _____

4) _____

64. Isopropyl alcohol and ethyl alcohol are both _____ alcohols.

65. Match each of the following chemical ingredients with its description.

_____ 1. Alkonolamines   a) Special type of oil used in hair conditioners

_____ 2. Ammonia   b) Sweet, colorless, oily substance

_____ 3. Glycerin   c) Substances used to neutralize acids or raise the pH of many hair products

_____ 4. Silicones   d) Contain carbon and evaporate very easily

_____ 5. Volatile organic   e) Colorless gas with a pungent odor
           compounds (VOCs)

66. The use of this chemical ingredient does not cause blackheads.

_____ a) Glycerin   _____ c) Ammonia

_____ b) Silicone   _____ d) VOCs

67. These ingredients evaporate very easily.

_____ a) Glycerins   _____ c) Alkonolamines

_____ b) Silicones   _____ d) VOCs

Understand Potential Hydrogen (pH) and How it Affects Hair, Skin, and Nails

68. What does pH stand for? _____

69. The term pH represents the quantity of _____.

70. A(n) _____ is an atom or molecule that carries an electrical charge.

71. _____ is the separation of an atom or molecule into positive and negative ions.

72. An ion with a negative electrical charge is a(n) _____; an ion with a positive electrical charge is a(n) _____.

73. Only products that contain water can have a pH.

_____ True   _____ False

74. What does the pH scale measure? _____

_____

75. The pH scale ranges from 0 to 14. Match each of the following pH values with the appropriate solution type.

_____ 1. pH below 7   a) Neutral solution

_____ 2. pH of 7   b) Acidic solution

_____ 3. pH above 7   c) Alkaline solution

76. The term _____ means multiples of 10.

77. A pH of 9 is how many more times more alkaline than a pH of 8?

_____ a) 10 times   _____ b) 100 times   _____ c) 1,000 times

78. Skin and hair have an average pH of:

_____ a) 4   _____ b) 5   _____ c) 6   _____ d) 7

79. Explain why pure water alone may be drying to the skin.

_____

_____

_____

80. All _____ owe their chemical reactivity to the hydrogen ion. Acids have a pH below _____.

81. An example of an acid that may be used in the salon is a(n) _____

_____.

82. Acids _____ and _____ the hair cuticle.

83. All _____ owe their chemical reactivity to the hydroxide ion. The terms _____ and _____ are interchangeable. Alkalis have a pH above _____.

84. Alkalis _____ and _____ hair, skin, the cuticle on the nail plate, and calloused skin.

85. Another term for sodium hydroxide is _____.

86. Name four safety precautions you should take when working with sodium hydroxide.

1) _____

2) _____

3) _____

4) _____

87. Acids and alkalis, when mixed together in equal proportions, create

_____.

88. Neutralizing shampoos and normalizing lotions used to neutralize hydroxide hair relaxers work by creating an acid-alkali _____ reaction.

89. Discuss one way to neutralize alkaline callous softener residues that may be left on a client's skin after rinsing.

_____

90. (W) **ACTIVITY:** Match each of the following terms with their identifying phrases, use, or definition.

Item Number	Term	Identifying Phrase, Use or Definition
_____	Anion	1. Subatomic particles with a negative charge
_____	Cation	2. Binds two or more incompatible materials into a fairly stable blend
_____	Chemical Change	3. Used in water-resistant lubricants for the skin
_____	Electron	4. Has a positive charge
_____	Emulsifier	5. Subatomic particles with a positive charge
_____	Glycolic acid	6. Has a strong, unpleasant odor
_____	Neutrons	7. Subatomic particles with no charge
_____	Protons	8. Has a negative charge
_____	Silicones	9. Used in exfoliation and to lower pH of products
_____	Thioglycolic acid	10. A change in the chemical composition or make-up of a substance

13 BASICS OF ELECTRICITY

Date: _____

Rating: _____

Text Pages: 272–291

why study BASICS OF ELECTRICITY?

1. List three reasons why a cosmetologist should study and have a thorough understanding of the basics of electricity.

   1) _____

   _____

   2) _____

   _____

   3) _____

   _____

   _____

Understand Electricity

2. _____ is the movement of electrons from one atom to another along a conductor.

3. When in motion, electricity exhibits _____, _____, or _____ effects.

4. A(n) _____ is the flow of electricity along a conductor.

5. Sparks are the visual form of electricity.

   _____ True   _____ False

6. Any material that allows electricity to pass through easily is a(n)

   _____.

7. Which of the following is a particularly good conductor?

   _____ a) Wood   _____ c) Cloth

   _____ b) Copper   _____ d) Alcohol

8. A material that does not transmit electricity is a(n) _____, also known as a(n) _____. Name five examples. _____

_____

9. Which of the following is not an insulator?

_____ a) Rubber _____ c) Cement

_____ b) Silk _____ d) Tap water

10. A(n) _____ Is the path of negative and positive electric currents moving from the generating source through the conductors and back to the generating source.

11. Name the two types of electric current.

1) _____

2) _____

12. _____ current is a constant, even-flowing current that travels in _____ direction and is produced by _____.

13. _____ current is a rapid and interrupted current, flowing first in one direction and then in the opposite direction.

14. What apparatus changes direct current to alternating current?

_____

15. What apparatus changes alternating current to direct current?

_____

16. Name which type of current each of the following items use.

a) Flashlights _____

b) Curling irons _____

c) Mobile phones _____

d) Table lamps _____

e) Car battery _____

f) Electric files _____

17. Match each term with its definition.

_____ 1. Volt a) Measures the strength of an electrical current

_____ 2. Ampere b) Measures how much electric energy is used in one second

_____ 3. Milliampere c) Equals 1,000 watts

_____ 4. Ohm   d) Measures the pressure or force that pushes electric current forward through a conductor

_____ 5. Watt   e) Equals one-thousandth of an ampere

_____ 6. Kilowatt   f) Measures the resistance of an electric current

Practice Electrical Equipment Safety

18. When electrical wires in a wall overheat, they could result in a(n)

_____.

19. A device that prevents excessive current from passing through a circuit is a(n)

_____.

20. A switch that automatically interrupts or shuts off an electric circuit at the first indication of overload is a(n) _____.

21. What does UL stand for? _____

22. What does the UL symbol mean when it is found on an electrical appliance?

_____

_____

23. What is grounding? _____

_____

24. List the 14 safety guidelines that you should adhere to when using electric appliances in the salon. The first guideline has been provided to get you started.

1) All of the electrical appliances used should be UL certified.

2) _____

3) _____

_____

4) _____

5) _____

6) _____

7) _____

_____

8) _____

_____

9) _____

_____

10) _____

11) _____

_____

12) _____

13) _____

14) _____

Understand Electrotherapy

25. The use of _____ to treat the skin is commonly referred to as electrotherapy.

26. Currents used in electrical _____ are called _____.

27. A(n) _____, or probe, is an applicator for directing electric current from an electrotherapy device to the client's skin and is usually made of _____, _____, or _____.

28. _____ is the negative or positive poles of an electric current. Electrodes on many electrotherapy devices have one positively charged pole, called a(n) _____, and one negatively charged pole, called a(n) _____.

29. The positive electrode is usually _____ and is marked with a *P* or a plus (+) sign.

30. The negative electrode is usually _____ and is marked with an *N* or minus (–) sign.

31. List the three modalities used in cosmetology.

1) _____

2) _____

3) _____

32. _____ current is a constant and direct current, having a positive and negative pole, that produces chemical changes when it passes through the tissues and fluids of the body.

33. The electrode used on the area to be treated is the _____ electrode; the _____ electrode is the opposite pole.

34. _____ is the process of infusing water-soluble products into the skin with the use of electric current.

35. _____ infuses an acidic product into deeper tissues using galvanic current from the positive pole toward the negative pole.

36. _____ infuses an alkaline product into the tissues from the negative pole toward the positive pole.

37. _____ is a process used to soften and emulsify grease deposits and blackheads in the hair follicles.

38. A client with pustular acne is a good candidate for receiving negative galvanic current.

    _____ True   _____ False

39. An extremely low level of electricity that mirrors the body's natural electrical impulses is called _____.

40. List nine ways this type of low-level electricity may be beneficial to clients.

    1) _____

    2) _____

    3) _____

    4) _____

    5) _____

    6) _____

    7) _____

    8) _____

    9) _____

41. The _____ is a thermal or heat-producing current with a high rate of oscillation or vibration that is commonly used for scalp and facial treatments; it is also known as _____.

42. The Tesla current electrodes are made from either _____ or _____.

43. List the five benefits from the use of Tesla high-frequency current.

1) _____

2) _____

3) _____

4) _____

5) _____

44. Neither Tesla high-frequency current nor microcurrent should be used on female patients who are _____.

Identify Other Electrical Equipment

45. Give the use or a description of each of the following electrical appliances.

a) Conventional hood hair dryers/heat lamps   _____

_____

b) Ionic hair dryers   _____

_____

c) Electric curling and flat irons   _____

_____

d) Heating caps   _____

_____

e) Haircolor processing machines   _____

_____

f) Steamers or vaporizers   _____

_____

g) Light therapy equipment   _____

_____

46. (W) **ACTIVITY:** In this chapter you have learned the importance of electricity in providing safe and effective cosmetology services. Think for a moment about how you are able to have electricity in your bathroom each morning in order for your blowdryer to operate. Ask yourself where the electricity comes from and what path it takes from its originating source to actually reach the on/off switch on the blow dryer. Using whatever tools you need (poster board, felt, construction paper, markers, rope, string, and so on) create a poster that depicts the journey electricity makes along the way. Get very creative and consider making the project three-dimensional (such as a mini-town). Internet research will be beneficial to make sure you capture every relevant step required in getting power to the people!

_____

_____

_____

_____

_____

_____

Explain Light Energy and Light Therapy

47. The electromagnetic spectrum is the name given to all of the forms of energy or _____ that exists.

48. The distance between successive peaks of electromagnetic waves is called the _____.

49. Long wavelengths have low frequency, meaning that the number of waves is _____ within a waveform pattern. Short wavelengths have higher frequency because the number of waves is _____ within a waveform pattern.

50. The _____ is the part of the electromagnetic spectrum that can be seen.

51. Visible light makes up only _____ of natural sunlight.

52. _____ and _____ are invisible because their wavelengths are beyond the visible spectrum of light. Combined they make up _____ of natural sunlight.

53. What are some other names for ultraviolet light? _____

_____

54. List six characteristics of ultraviolet light.

    1) _____

    2) _____

    3) _____

    4) _____

    5) _____

    6) _____

    7) _____

    8) _____

    9) _____

55. Which of the following types of UV light is often used in tanning beds?

    _____ a) UVA   _____ b) UVB   _____ c) UVC

56. _____ has longer wavelengths, penetrates more deeply, has less energy, and produces more heat than visible light. It make up _____ percent of natural sunlight.

57. What are some uses for infrared light in the salon? _____

    _____

    _____

    _____

58. _____ are substances that speed up chemical reactions. Some use _____ as an energy source while others use

    _____.

59. What is light therapy? _____

    _____

60. What does the acronym LASER stand for?

    L: _____

    A: _____

    S: _____

    E: _____

    R: _____

61. What does the process of photothermolysis do? _____

_____

62. What does LED stand for?

L: _____

E: _____

D: _____

63. Which color LED reduces acne? _____

64. Which color LED increases circulation and improves collagen and elastin production in the skin? _____

65. Which color LED reduces swelling and inflammation? _____

66. What is the name of a medical device that uses multiple colors and wavelengths of focused light to treat spider veins, hyperpigmentation, rosacea and redness, wrinkles, enlarged hair follicles and pores, and excessive hair?

_____

14 PRINCIPLES OF HAIR DESIGN

Date: _____

Rating: _____

Text Pages: 294–319

why study PRINCIPLES OF HAIR DESIGN?

1. An understanding of design and _____ will help you develop the artistic skill and judgment needed to create the best possible design for your client.

2. By having a better understanding of the principles of hair design, you will: understand why a particular hairstyle will or will not be the _____ for a client; have helpful guidelines to assist in achieving your _____; be able to create haircuts and styles designed to help clients _____ areas of concern while _____ their most attractive areas.

Discover the Philosophy of Design

3. Modern inspiration in fashion often starts as _____ which then moves to the streets as a phenomenon or trend.

4. List some sources of inspiration. _____

_____

5. One of the best sources of design inspiration can be found in _____

_____.

6. What places, things, or people inspire your creativity?

_____

_____

7. A good designer always envisions the end result before beginning.

_____ True   _____ False

8. Once inspired, what do you need to decide next?

_____

9. You have been inspired by a photograph and want to try out a new design. When working out the details and planning of a design, where should you begin?

_____ a) On your next client   _____ b) On yourself   _____ c) On a mannequin head

10. As a designer, what must you develop? _____

_____

11. Along with learning through study, it is best to _____ until you gain a working knowledge of the process of hair design.

12. Having a strong foundation in technique along with practicing personal skills will allow you to take _____.

13. Often stylists limit positive risks and confine themselves to their current comfort zone. Sometimes comfort zones can translate into:

_____ a) "risk-taker."

_____ b) "outside-the-box innovator."

_____ c) "dated and uninspiring."

14. Great hairstylists find inspiration everywhere by keeping an eye out for what is new in the beauty industry and be dedicating themselves to their _____

_____.

Define the Elements of Hair Design

15. What are the five basic elements of three-dimensional design?

1) _____   4) _____

2) _____   5) _____

3) _____

16. _____ define form and space and create the shape, design, and movement of a hairstyle. They can be _____ or _____.

17. Match each of the four basic types of lines with its description.

_____ 1. Horizontal lines   a) Lines are up and down

_____ 2. Vertical lines   b) Lines moving in a circular or semicircular direction

_____ 3. Diagonal lines   c) Positioned between horizontal and vertical lines

_____ 4. Curved lines   d) Extend in the same direction and maintain a constant distance apart and are parallel from the floor and relative to the horizon

18. Describe the usage of the basic types of lines.

a) Horizontal lines _____

_____

b) Vertical lines _____

_____

c) Diagonal lines _____

_____

d) Curved lines _____

_____

19. A client would like a hairstyle that minimizes her large nose. Which type of line might be most helpful in a design to meet this goal? _____

20. Describe a **single line** in hairstyling. _____

_____

_____

21. Describe a **parallel line** in hairstyling. _____

_____

_____

22. Describe a **contrasting line** in hairstyling. _____

_____

_____

23. Describe a **transitional line** in hairstyling. _____

_____

_____

24. Describe a **directional line** in hairstyling. _____

_____

_____

25. _____ is a mass or general outline of a hairstyle that is three-dimensional and has _____, _____, and _____.

26. Form may also be referred to as _____.

27. Solid, smoother forms with minimal texture most often give a(n) _____ appearance to the outline of the style, where more textured forms can add _____.

28. The hair form should be in proportion to the:

a) _____

b) _____

c) _____

29. _____ is the area surrounding the form or the area the hairstyle occupies and may contain _____, _____, _____, _____, or any combination.

30. We are more aware of the _____ form than the _____ spaces.

31. The directional wave patterns or _____ must be taken into consideration when creating a style for your client.

32. All hair has a unique directional pattern described as:

a) _____

b) _____

c) _____

d) _____

33. Choose one (or more) of the natural wave patterns identified in the previous question to complete the following.

a) These types of wave patterns can create a larger form. _____

b) This type of wave pattern reflects light better. _____

c) This type can be combed directionally to create horizontal lines. _____

34. How can texture be created temporarily? _____

_____

35. List 10 techniques or tools that will temporarily change hair texture.

1) _____

2) _____

3) _____

4) _____

5) _____

6) _____

7) _____

8) _____

9) _____

10) _____

36. How can texture be changed permanently? _____

_____

37. How long does a permanent texture change last?

_____

38. When is it appropriate to use multiple directional wave pattern combinations together?

_____

_____

39. _____ wave patterns accent the face and are particularly useful when you wish to narrow a round head shape.

40. _____ wave patterns take attention away from the face and can be used to soften square or rectangular features.

41. What two roles does haircolor play in hair design?

a) _____

b) _____

42. Discuss why you think that haircolor is important to the client psychologically in the overall look of a hair design.

_____

_____

_____

_____

_____

_____

43. _____ can be used to make all or part of the design appear larger or smaller and can help define _____ and _____.

44. Light and warm colors create the illusion of _____.

45. _____ and _____ colors recede or move in toward the head, creating the illusion of less volume.

46. Explain how to create the illusion of dimension or depth.

_____

_____

_____

47. Using a _____ color will draw a line in the hairstyle in the direction you want the eye to travel.

48. How can you use color to create a bold, dramatic accent?

_____

49. What should be considered when choosing a color?

_____

_____

_____

50. For a client with a gold tone to her skin, _____ haircolors are more flattering.

_____ cool   _____ warm

51. High contrast colors work best for a conservative look.

_____ True   _____ False

Understand the Principles of Hair Design

52. The five principles for art and design of hair design are:

1) _____

2) _____

3) _____

4) _____

5) _____

53. Match each of the following principles of art and design with its description.

_____ 1. Proportion   a) Where the eye is drawn to first; also known as focus

_____ 2. Balance   b) Creation of unity in a design; the most important of the art principles

_____ 3. Rhythm   c) Establishing equal or appropriate proportions to create symmetry

_____ 4. Emphasis   d) Regular pulsation or recurrent pattern of movement in a design

_____ 5. Harmony   e) Comparative relationship of one thing to another

54. When designing a hairstyle, it is essential that you take into account the client's

_____.

55. What style would you normally create for a woman with large hips or broad shoulders? _____ Explain your answer:

_____

56. What is the general guide for classic proportion? _____

_____

_____

57. Which element of design can be either symmetrical or asymmetrical?

_____

58. Explain how to measure symmetry. _____

_____

_____

59. Describe symmetrical balance. _____

_____

_____

_____

60. Describe asymmetrical balance. _____

_____

_____

_____

61. Define *rhythm* in a design. _____

_____

62. Which of the following signifies a fast rhythm?

_____ a) Tight curls   _____ b) Loose curls

63. What is meant by emphasis in a design?

_____

_____

64. List four options you may choose to create an area of emphasis or focus in a hairstyle.

1) _____

2) _____

3) _____

4) _____

65. A hair design should have only one point or area of emphasis.

_____ True   _____ False

66. Explain the importance of harmony in a hair design.

_____

67. When a hairstyle is harmonious, it contains what three elements?

1) _____

2) _____

3) _____

68. A successful harmonious design includes an area of emphasis.

_____ True   _____ False

69. The best results are obtained when each of your client's facial features and profile is properly analyzed for its _____ and _____.

70. An artistic and suitable hairstyle will take into account the following physical characteristics of the client:

a) _____

b) _____

c) _____

d) _____

Recognize the Influence of Hair Type and Texture on Hairstyle

71. Your client's hair type is a major consideration in the selection of a hairstyle. What are the two defining characteristics to consider?

_____

72. List the three basic types of hair texture.

1) _____

2) _____

3) _____

73. Match each of the following hair textures with its description.

_____ 1. Straight, fine hair   a) Offers the most versatility in styling

_____ 2. Straight, medium hair   b) Hard to curl; responds well to thermal styling with flat tools

_____ 3. Straight, coarse hair   c) Often separates, revealing the client's scalp

_____ 4. Wavy, fine hair   d) Generally best cut short

_____ 5. Wavy, medium hair   e) When left natural gives a soft, romantic look

_____ 6. Wavy, coarse hair   f) Tends to widen as it grows longer

_____ 7. Curly, fine hair   g) Hugs the head shape due to lack of body or volume

_____ 8. Curly, medium hair   h) May appear fuller when diffused with heat and the appropriate haircut and style

_____ 9. Curly, coarse hair   i) Will be extremely wide, often appears dense, offers limited flexibility

_____ 10. Very curly, fine hair   j) Usually very compacted with little to no movement

_____ 11. Extremely curly, medium hair   k) Can produce a voluminous silhouette if not shaped properly

_____ 12. Extremely curly, coarse hair   l) Offers more versatility in styling; good amount of movement

Create Harmony Between Hairstyle and Facial Structure

74. A client's facial shape is determined by the _____ and _____ of the facial bones.

75. What is the best way to determine a client's facial shape?

_____

_____

76. List the seven basic facial shapes.

1) _____

2) _____

3) _____

4) _____

5) _____

6) _____

7) _____

77. When designing a style for your client's facial type, you generally are trying to create the illusion of a(n) _____ face shape.

78. To determine a facial shape, divide the face into _____ zones. They are

_____

_____.

79. Describe the facial contour of the oval face. _____

_____

_____

80. What type of hairstyle works best on a client with an oval face?

_____

_____

81. Describe the facial contour, the objective, and the styling choice for the **round** facial type.

Facial contour: _____

_____

Objective: _____

_____

Styling choice: _____

_____

82. Describe the facial contour, the objective, and the styling choice for the **square** facial type.

Facial contour: _____

_____

Objective: _____

_____

Styling choice: _____

_____

83. Describe the facial contour, the objective, and the styling choice for the **triangular** (pear-shaped) facial type.

Facial contour: _____

_____

Objective: _____

_____

Styling choice: _____

_____

84. Describe the facial contour, the objective, and the styling choice for the **oblong** facial type.

Facial contour: _____

Objective: _____

Styling choice: _____

_____

85. Describe the facial contour, the objective, and the styling choice for the **diamond** facial type.

Facial contour: _____

_____

Objective: _____

_____

Styling choice: _____

_____

86. Describe the facial contour, the objective, and the styling choice for the **inverted triangle** (heart-shaped) facial type.

Facial contour: _____

Objective: _____

_____

Styling choice: _____

_____

_____

_____

87. A long hairstyle is not usually recommended for a client with a(n) _____ facial type.

_____ a) inverted triangle   _____ c) oblong

_____ b) square   _____ d) oval

88. Bangs are often recommended in hairstyles for clients who have a(n) _____ facial type.

_____ a) inverted triangle   _____ c) oblong

_____ b) square   _____ d) oval

89. The _____ is the outline of the face, head, or figure seen in a side view.

90. Match each of the following basic profiles with its description.

_____ 1. Straight   a) Has a prominent forehead and chin

_____ 2. Convex   b) Considered ideal; has a very slight curvature

_____ 3. Concave   c) Has a receding forehead and chin

91. This profile type looks best with hairstyles that include an arrangement of bangs or curls over the forehead. _____

92. This profile type looks best when the hair at the nape of the neck is styled with an upward movement. _____

93. How should you style the hair for a wide forehead?

_____

94. How should you style the hair for a narrow forehead?

_____

95. A large forehead looks best with bangs that have a large amount of volume.

_____ True _____ False

96. How should you style the hair for close-set eyes?

_____

_____

97. The hair should be slightly lighter at the sides than at the top for wide-set eyes.

_____ True _____ False

98. How should you style the hair for wide-set eyes?

_____

99. How should you style the hair for a crooked nose?

_____

100. How should you style the hair for a wide, flat nose?

_____

_____

101. How should you style the hair for a long, narrow nose?

_____

_____

102. A hairstyle with a middle part is a poor choice for a client who has a long, narrow nose.

_____ True _____ False

103. Provide the correct styling tip for the following facial features.

a) Round jaw: _____

_____

b) Square jaw: _____

_____

c) Long jaw: _____

_____

d) Receding forehead: _____

_____

e) Large forehead: _____

_____

f) Small nose: _____

_____

g) Prominent nose: _____

_____

h) Receding chin: _____

_____

i) Small chin: _____

_____

j) Large chin: _____

_____

104. How should you style the hair for a head that is not completely round?

_____

_____

105. What is a major consideration when creating a hairstyle for someone who wears glasses?

_____

_____

106. Where is the bang or fringe area located?

_____

_____

107. List the three ways that the bang area or fringe can be parted.

1) _____

2) _____

3) _____

108. List the four partings that can be used to highlight facial features.

1) _____

2) _____

3) _____

4) _____

109. Choose the correct parting type from the list above to complete the following.

a) This can help make thin hair appear fuller: _____.

b) This gives an oval illusion to wide and round faces: _____.

c) This is used to create a dramatic effect: _____.

d) This can help create an illusion of width or height: _____.

110. ACTIVITY: Look through old magazines or on the Internet for pictures of celebrities. Select at least six pictures focusing on head shots of both males and females. Cut out the pictures and place them on a poster board or mount them on card stock and place them in a binder. Using the following format, complete the information for each photograph and place the information with the photograph on the poster or in the binder. Be creative and make your presentation of information professional in appearance.

Face Shape.

Styling Objective for the Face Shape.

Was the styling achieved in the style selected?

If not, what should have been done differently?

Describe which types of lines were used in the style (vertical, horizontal, diagonal, curved).

Describe the proportion used in the hairstyle.

State where the area of emphasis is in the style.

Describe how the rhythm, harmony, and balance were employed (or not).

Is the style symmetrical or asymmetrical and explain your answer.

If you could create another style for this celebrity, what would it be and why?

_____

_____

_____

_____

_____

_____

_____

Design for Men

111. As a professional, what types of styles should you recommend for a man?

_____

_____

112. Men are limited to only a few hairstyle options.

_____ True   _____ False

113. Mustaches, beards, and sideburns can be a great way for a male client to show his individual style and _____.

114. A man who is balding with closely trimmed hair could look very good in a closely groomed _____.

Date: _____

Rating: _____

Text Pages: 320–355

1. One of the most important experiences that a stylist provides is the

   _____.

2. The shampoo service actually encompasses three different processes: _____

   _____, _____, and _____.

3. The shampoo can and should be:

   a) _____

   b) _____

why study SCALP CARE, SHAMPOOING AND CONDITIONING?

4. List four reasons a cosmetologist should study and have a thorough understanding of scalp care, shampooing, and conditioning.

   1) _____

   _____

   2) _____

   _____

   3) _____

   4) _____

   _____

Safely And Effectively Use Massage in Scalp Care

5. List the two basic requirements for a healthy scalp.

   1) _____

   2) _____

6. How often should the hair be shampooed?   _____

   _____

7. The same products are used for both relaxation and treatment massages.

   _____ True   _____ False

8. The manipulations for a treatment massage mirror those of a relaxation massage but would include the _____.

9. A client who has high blood pressure should never have a scalp massage.

   _____ True   _____ False

   Explain your answer: _____

   _____

   _____

   _____

10. If you are unsure about whether it would be appropriate to perform a scalp massage on a client who has a medical condition, the best course would be to:

   _____ a) avoid performing the massage.

   _____ b) assume it is fine since the client does not have a doctor's note.

   _____ c) skip the shampoo service.

11. List the four different types of scalp treatments.

   1) _____

   2) _____

   3) _____

   4) _____

12. Complete the following by listing the appropriate type of scalp treatment.

    a) This may be done in combination with a scalp steamer: _____

    _____

    b) The main goal of this treatment is to maintain the scalp and hair in a clean and

    healthy condition: _____

    c) A client may need additional salon treatments and the frequent use of home

    care: _____

    d) This treatment is performed for clients who have overactive sebaceous glands:

    _____

13. Dandruff is caused by a _____ called _____.

Learn the Benefits of Proper Hair Brushing

14. List three benefits of correct hair brushing.

    1) _____

    2) _____

    3) _____

15. Do not brush a client's hair if it is oily.

    _____ True   _____ False

16. List at least three situations under which brushing a client's hair should be avoided.

    1) _____

    2) _____

    3) _____

    4) _____

17. The best type of hairbrush to use for brushing hair is one that has _____ bristles.

    _____ a) natural   _____ b) plastic   _____ c) nylon

Provide A Proper and Effective Shampoo Service

18. The shampoo service provides a good opportunity to make sure that the hair and scalp are properly cleansed and nourished, providing a great _____ for styling and ongoing hair care.

19. What conditions should you check for when analyzing the scalp and hair?

    a) _____

    b) _____

    c) _____

    d) _____

    e) _____

    f) _____

    g) _____

    h) _____

    i) _____

20. You should not perform a scalp massage on a scalp that has reddened scalp irritations.

    _____ True   _____ False

21. A client appears to have a scalp disease that may be infectious. What should you do?

    _____

    _____

22. The primary purpose of a shampoo is to _____ the hair and scalp prior to a service.

23. To be effective, a shampoo must _____

    _____.

24. You should advise all clients to wash their hair every day.

    _____ True   _____ False

25. What does excessive shampooing do? _____

    _____

    _____

26. Oily hair should be shampooed more often than normal or dry hair.

_____ True   _____ False

27. Describe two ways you can help protect yourself from muscle strain and other physical problems that may be caused by performing shampoos on clients.

1) _____

_____

2) _____

_____

28. Professional cosmetologists should take time to read product _____ because doing this will help them make informed decisions about the use of various shampoos.

29. How should you select a shampoo for a client? _____

_____

30. Hair can usually be characterized as:

a) _____

b) _____

c) _____

d) _____

31. Hair that has been _____ may require a product, such as a(n) _____ shampoo, that is less harsh and more conditioning.

32. Hair that has been damaged by improper care and exposure to _____ such as wind, sun, cold, and heat may need to be treated with more conditioning agents.

33. List four examples of ways hair may be chemically treated.

1) _____

2) _____

3) _____

4) _____

34. List three ways hair may be damaged.

1) _____

2) _____

3) _____

35. As long as clients look great when they leave the salon, how they handle their home-care regimen is unimportant to you as a professional.

_____ True   _____ False

Explain your answer: _____

_____

_____

_____

36. Discuss why it is important to educate clients about which products they should be using for home care. _____

_____

_____

37. The amount of _____ in a solution is what determines whether it is alkaline or acid.

38. A pH scale ranges from:

_____ a) 0–8   _____ c) 0–14

_____ b) 0–12   _____ d) 0–18

39. A neutral shampoo has a pH of _____.

40. A shampoo that is _____ will have a pH ranging from 0 to 6.9.

41. A shampoo that is _____ will have a pH rating of 7.1 or higher.

42. The _____ the pH rating, the stronger and harsher the shampoo.

43. A slightly _____ shampoo more closely matches the ideal pH of hair.

44. Why should you avoid touching a female client's face with your hands or water while performing a shampoo?

_____

_____

45. It is easy to miss which of the following when performing a shampoo?

_____ a) The bang area   _____ c) The top of the head

_____ b) Behind the ears   _____ d) The nape of the neck

46. Water is classified as a(n) _____ because it is capable of dissolving more substances than any other solvent known to science.

47. Water that comes from a public water system often has _____ added to it to kill _____.

48. The process of heating water so that it becomes a vapor and then condensing the purified vapor so that it collects as a liquid is called _____.

49. _____ is rainwater or chemically softened water.

50. _____ is often found in well water and contains minerals that reduce the ability of soap or shampoo to lather.

51. Why is it important for you to understand the classification of the water in the salon

where you work? _____

_____

52. Water is the main ingredient in most shampoos.

_____ True   _____ False

53. What is deionized water? _____

_____

_____

54. Primary surfactant and base detergent mean the same thing as follows: _____

_____.

55. A surfactant molecule has two ends: a _____ "head," and a _____ "tail."

56. During the shampoo process, the hydrophilic head attracts _____ and the lipophilic tail attracts _____.

57. What does the process create? _____

_____

_____

58. List six ingredients that may be added to base surfactants to create a shampoo.

1. _____   4. _____

2. _____   5. _____

3. _____   6. _____

59. Match each type of shampoo with its purpose.

_____ 1. pH-balanced shampoos   a) Contain special ingredients that are very effective in reducing dandruff or relieving other scalp conditions

_____ 2. Conditioning shampoos   b) Wash away excess oiliness, while preventing the hair from drying out

_____ 3. Medicated shampoos   c) Designed to make the hair appear smooth and shiny

_____

4. Clarifying shampoos   d) Used to brighten, to add a slight hint of color, or to eliminate unwanted color tones

_____ 5. Balancing shampoos   e) Special solutions available for hair enhancements

_____ 6. Dry or powder shampoos   f) Balanced to the pH of skin and hair

_____ 7. Color-enhancing shampoos   g) Cleanse the hair without the use of soap and water

_____ 8. Shampoos for hairpieces and wigs   h) Used when product build up is evident, after swimming, and prior to all chemical services

60. How should you shampoo a client who is in a wheelchair?

_____

_____

_____

_____

_____

61. (W) **ACTIVITY:** Request permission to evaluate the labels of all the shampoos used in the institution. Further the experiment by bringing in the bottles of shampoo used in your home. Make a list of all the products, and then list their top four ingredients. Evaluate which ingredients are common among all the products. Research what those ingredients do and explain why each particular ingredient is beneficial to hair. Use the format below to document your findings.

Product	Top Four Ingredients* (*Notates the Common Ingredients)	Purpose
TRESemmé	Water*	The universal solvent
	Sodium Laureth Sulfate*	Effective foaming agent
	Cocamidopropyl Betaine*	Surfactant used as a foam booster
	Sodium Chloride	Salt is a cleansing agent
Suave® for Men	Water*	The universal solvent
	Sodium Laureth Sulfate*	Effective foaming agent
	Cocamidopropyl Betaine*	Surfactant used as a foam booster
	Dimethiconol	Silicone based hair conditioning agent

Recommend and Use Conditioners

62. _____ are special chemical agents applied to the hair to deposit protein or moisturizer, to help restore the hair's strength, to infuse moisture, to give it body, or to protect it against possible breakage.

63. Conditioners can fully repair hair and can improve the quality of new hair growth.

_____ True _____ False

64. What are the four basic types of conditioners?

1) _____

2) _____

3) _____

4) _____

65. What are humectants? _____

_____

66. Why is silicone often added to conditioners? _____

_____

67. Explain what conditioners do. _____

_____

68. The cortex accounts for what percentage of the hair strand?

_____ a) 25 percent   _____ c) 75 percent

_____ b) 60 percent   _____ d) 90 percent

69. _____ are designed to penetrate the cortex and reinforce the hair shaft from within to temporarily reconstructing the hair.

70. List and describe four additional conditioning agents to be familiar with.

1) _____

_____

2) _____

_____

3) _____

_____

4) _____

_____

71. A client who has coarse and extremely curly hair would benefit most from which of the following products?

_____ a) Volumizing shampoo

_____ b) Protein and moisturizing treatments

_____ c) Spray-on thermal protection

_____ d) pH/acid balanced shampoo

72. A client who has straight, fine hair would benefit most from which of the following products?

_____ a) Leave-in conditioner   _____ c) Finishing rinse

_____ b) Moisturizing treatments   _____ d) Volumizing shampoo

73. _____, also known as hair masks or conditioning packs, are chemical mixtures of concentrated protein and intensive moisturizer.

Use Professional Draping

74. List the two types of draping that are used on clients.

1) _____

2) _____

75. Describe why you think it is important for you to learn how to drape a client properly.

_____

_____

_____

_____

_____

_____

_____

Understand the Benefits of the Three-Part Procedure

76. The stylist preparation portion of the pre-service procedure includes, among other things, reviewing the appointment schedule and resolving any potential time conflicts, retrieving the client's intake form and service record card, reviewing them, _____ yourself, turning off your _____, taking a moment to clear your head of all personal concerns and issues, and washing your hands thoroughly before going to greet your client.

77. Describe the objective of the postservice procedure.

_____

_____

_____

_____

_____

CHAPTER *16* # HAIRCUTTING

See Milady Standard Cosmetology Practical Workbook.

CHAPTER *17* # HAIRSTYLING

See Milady Standard Cosmetology Practical Workbook.

CHAPTER *18* # BRAIDING & BRAID EXTENSIONS

See Milady Standard Cosmetology Practical Workbook.

CHAPTER *19* # WIGS & HAIR ADDITIONS

See Milady Standard Cosmetology Practical Workbook.

20 CHEMICAL TEXTURE SERVICES

Date: _____

Rating: _____

Text Pages: 596–667

why study CHEMICAL TEXTURE SERVICES?

1. Texture services can be used to _____ straight hair, _____ overly curly hair, or _____ tightly coiled hair.

2. List the reasons a cosmetologist who performs chemical texture services should study and have a basic understanding of chemical texture services.

   a) _____

   _____

   b) _____

   _____

   c) _____

   _____

   d) _____

   _____

   e) _____

   _____

3. _____ services are hair services that cause a chemical change within the hair's natural wave and curl pattern.

4. Chemical textures services include:

   a) _____

   _____

b) _____

_____

c) _____

_____

Understand How Chemical Services Affect the Structure of Hair

5. The _____ layer is the tough exterior layer of the hair. It surrounds the inner layers and _____ the hair from damage.

6. The cuticle is directly involved in the texture or movement of the hair.

_____ True   _____ False

7. The _____ is the middle layer of the hair, located directly beneath the _____ layer.

8. The cortex is responsible for the incredible _____ and _____ of human hair.

9. _____ the side bonds of the _____ makes it possible to change the natural wave pattern of the hair.

10. The _____ is often called the pith or core of the hair and does not play a role in chemical texture services.

11. Fine hair may not contain which of the following parts?

_____ a) Cuticle   _____ b) Cortex   _____ c) Medulla

12. What does the term *pH* mean? _____

13. What does the pH scale measure?

_____

14. An acidic substance has a pH _____.

15. An alkaline substance has a pH _____.

16. What is the natural pH of hair? _____

17. Explain what chemical solutions do to change the hair's natural curl pattern.

_____

_____

_____

18. Coarse, resistant hair with a strong, compact cuticle layer requires a highly acidic chemical solution.

_____ True   _____ False

19. Match each term related to the basic building block of hair with its definition.

_____ 1. Amino acids

a) Long chains of amino acids joined together by peptide bonds

_____ 2. Peptide bonds

b) Cross-linked polypeptide chains

_____ 3. Polypeptide chains

c) Compounds made up of carbon, oxygen, hydrogen, nitrogen, and sulfur

_____ 4. Keratin proteins

d) Weak physical side bonds that are the result of an attraction between opposite electrical charges

_____ 5. Side bonds

e) Relatively weak physical side bonds that are the result of an attraction between negative and positive electrical charges

_____ 6. Disulfide bonds

f) Chemical side bonds formed when the sulfur atoms in two adjacent protein chains are joined together

_____ 7. Salt bonds

g) Long, coiled polypeptide chains

_____ 8. Hydrogen bonds

h) End bonds; join amino acids together end-to-end in long chains

20. Which type of bond is the strongest of the three side bonds?

_____

21. How are salt bonds broken? _____

Demonstrate the Proper Technique for Permanent Waving

22. What are the two steps of the permanent wave process?

1) _____

_____

2) _____

_____

23. It is important to do an elasticity test before perming the hair.

_____ True   _____ False

24. What do alkaline permanent waving solutions do?

_____

_____

25. Once the waving solution is in the cortex, what occurs?

_____

_____

26. What is a reduction reaction?

_____

_____

27. What is a reduction reaction in permanent waving?

_____

_____

28. Explain the four steps in the chemical process of permanent waving.

1) _____

_____

_____

2) _____

_____

_____

3) _____

_____

_____

4) _____

_____

_____

29. What is the reducing agent used in permanent waving solutions?

_____

_____

_____

30. _____ is the most common reducing agent in permanent wave solutions.

31. The strength of the permanent waving solution is determined primarily by

_____.

32. Why is ammonia added to the thioglycolic acid product?

_____

_____

33. The addition of ammonia to thioglycolic acid produces a new chemical called

_____ which is alkaline and is the active ingredient or reducing agent in alkaline permanents.

34. Which type of hair will need a more alkaline solution to achieve permanent waving?

_____

35. Another name for alkaline waves is _____.

36. Alkaline waves have a pH between _____.

37. _____ is the main active ingredient in true acid and acid-balanced waving lotions.

38. What are the three separate components of all acid waves?

1) _____

2) _____

3) _____

39. The first _____ were introduced in the early 1970s and have a pH between _____. They require heat to process.

40. Most of the acid waves found in today's salons have a pH between:

_____ a) 5.8 and 6.2.   _____ c) 7.8 and 8.2.

_____ b) 6.8 and 7.2.   _____ d) 8.8 and 9.2.

41. _____ process at room temperature, do not require the added heat of a hair dryer, process more quickly, and produce firmer curls than true acid waves.

42. _____ create a chemical reaction that heats up the waving solution and speeds up the processing.

43. What are the three components of exothermic waves?

1) _____

2) _____

3) _____

44. When creating exothermic waves, mixing an oxidizer with permanent waving solution causes _____

_____.

45. _____ are activated by an outside heat source, usually a conventional hood-type hair dryer.

46. _____ use an ingredient that does not evaporate as readily as ammonia, so there is very little odor associated with their use.

47. Ammonia-free waves will not damage hair, even if used incorrectly.

_____ True   _____ False

48. Where can information about the ingredients, strength, and pH of permanent wave solutions be found?

_____

49. _____ use an ingredient other than ATG, such as cysteamine or mercaptamine, as the primary reducing agent.

50. The use of sulfates, sulfites, and bisulfites present an alternative to ATG known as

_____.

51. Sulfite permanents are usually marketed as _____

_____.

52. The strength of any permanent wave is based on the concentration of its

_____.

53. The amount of processing during a permanent wave is determined by the _____ of the permanent waving solution.

54. In permanent waving, most of the processing takes place as soon as the solution _____.

55. What does the additional processing time allow?

_____

56. When does overprocessing usually occur?

_____

57. Resistant hair may not become completely saturated with just one application of waving solution.

_____ True   _____ False

58. To achieve curlier hair, always process it longer.

_____ True   _____ False

59. What occurs if the hair is underprocessed? _____

_____

60. _____ stops the action of the waving solution and rebuilds the hair into its new curly form.

61. What are the two important functions of neutralization?

1) _____

2) _____

62. The most common neutralizer is _____.

63. Oxidative reactions can _____ hair color, especially at an alkaline pH.

64. When rinsing perm solution from hair, how long should you rinse?

_____

65. If the hair is insufficiently blotted, what will occur?

_____

66. When rinsing the hair, you should always use hot water.

_____ True   _____ False

67. When rinsing the hair, use a gentle stream of water.

_____ True   _____ False

68. Always _____ the hair after the recommended rinsing time.

69. How should you towel-blot the hair after rinsing?

_____

70. Always adjust any rods that have become _____ prior to applying the neutralizer.

71. _____ breaks disulfide bonds by adding hydrogen. _____ rebuilds the disulfide bonds by removing the hydrogen that was added by the permanent waving solution.

72. What information do you obtain from preliminary test curls?

a) _____

_____

b) _____

_____

c) _____

_____

d) _____

_____

e) _____

_____

f) _____

_____

g) _____

_____

73. _____ are the most common type of perm rod. They have a smaller _____ in the center that increases to a larger diameter on the ends.

74. _____ are equal in diameter along their entire length or curling area.

75. Concave rods produce a _____ in the center, and a _____ on either side of the strand.

76. Straight rods produce a(n) _____ along the entire width of the strand.

77. _____ are usually about 12 inches (30.5 cm) long with a uniform diameter along the entire length of the rod.

78. What allows these soft foam roads to bend into almost any shape?

_____

79. The _____ or _____ rod is usually about 12 inches (30.5 cm) long with a uniform diameter along the entire length of the rod.

80. What does perming only the base of the hair achieve?

_____

81. _____ are thin, absorbent papers used to control the ends of the hair when wrapping and winding hair on the perm rods.

82. What is another name for the answer to #81? _____

83. Why is it important to extend end papers beyond the ends of the hair?

_____

84. List the three most common end paper techniques and explain each.

1) _____

_____

2) _____

_____

3) _____

_____

85. All perm wraps begin by sectioning the hair into _____.

86. How do you determine the size, shape, and direction of panels?

_____

_____

87. Each panel is divided into subsections called _____.

88. _____ refers to the position of the rod in relation to its base section, and it is determined by the angle at which the hair is wrapped.

89. Rods can be wrapped in three ways as follows:

1) _____

2) _____

3) _____

90. For on-base placement, the hair is wrapped _____ beyond perpendicular to its base section.

91. Half off-base placement refers to wrapping the hair at an angle of _____ or perpendicular to its base section.

92. Half off-base placement _____ stress and tension on the hair.

93. Off-base placement refers to wrapping the hair at _____ below the center of the base section.

94. Which placement creates the least amount of volume and results in curl patterns that begin farthest away from the scalp? _____

95. Base direction refers to the angle at which the rod is positioned on the head:
_____, _____, or _____.

96. Why is it important to remember to wrap in the natural direction of hair growth?

_____

97. What are the two methods of wrapping the hair around the perm rod?

1) _____

2) _____

98. In which wrapping method is the hair strand wound around the rod, going from the ends to the scalp? _____

99. Which wrapping method produces a uniform curl from the scalp to ends?

_____

100. Which wrapping method produces tighter curl at the ends, and a larger curl at the scalp? _____

101. What is a double-rod or piggyback wrap?

_____

_____

102. What is the benefit of wrapping hair in a piggyback wrap?

_____

_____

103. List six wrapping patterns that are used in permanent waving.

1) _____

2) _____

3) _____

4) _____

5) _____

6) _____

104. Your client would like more volume in one specific area. What solution might you recommend? _____

105. Permanent waving a man's hair requires the use of different techniques than perming a woman's hair.

_____ True   _____ False

106. List the safety precautions for permanent waving. The first precaution is listed to help you get started.

a) Protect the client's clothing.

b) _____

_____

c) _____

_____

d) _____

_____

e) _____

_____

f) _____

_____

g) _____

_____

h) _____

_____

i) _____

_____

j) _____

_____

k) _____

_____

l) _____

_____

m) _____

_____

n) _____

_____

107. Some home haircoloring products contain _____ that are not compatible with permanent waving.

Demonstrate the Proper Technique for Chemical Hair Relaxers

108. _____ is the process of rearranging the structure of curly hair into a straighter or smoother form.

109. The chemistry of relaxers and permanent waving is exactly the same.

_____ True   _____ False

110. The most common types of chemical hair relaxers are _____, _____, and _____.

111. Extremely curly hair grows in long twisted spirals or coils, with the thinnest and weakest sections of the hair strands located at their twists.

_____ True   _____ False

112. _____ use the same ATG that is used in permanent waving but at a higher concentration and a higher pH.

113. A relaxer can melt hair if it is used incorrectly.

_____ True   _____ False

114. The _____ used with thio relaxers is an oxidizing agent, usually hydrogen peroxide, just as in permanents.

115. _____ combines use of a thio relaxer with a flat iron.

116. The _____ is the active ingredient in all hydroxide relaxers.

117. Hydroxide relaxers are very strong alkalis that can swell the hair up to twice its normal diameter.

_____ True   _____ False

118. Why are hydroxide relaxers not compatible with thio relaxers, permanent waves, or soft curl perms? _____

119. In _____, the process by which hydroxide relaxers permanently straighten hair, the relaxers remove a sulfur atom from a disulfide bond, converting it into a lanthionine bond.

120. Hair that has been treated with a _____ is unfit for permanent waving and will not hold a curl.

121. _____ are ionic compounds formed by a metal—sodium (Na), potassium (K), or lithium (Li)—which is combined with oxygen (O) and hydrogen (H).

122. Sodium hydroxide (NaOH) relaxers are commonly called _____

_____.

123. _____ and _____ relaxers are often advertised and sold as "no mix—no lye" relaxers.

124. _____ relaxers are also advertised and sold as no-lye relaxers.

125. Guanidine hydroxide relaxers straighten the hair completely, with less scalp irritation than other hydroxide relaxers.

_____ True   _____ False

126. _____ and _____ are sometimes used as low-pH hair relaxers.

127. _____ is an oily cream used to protect the skin and scalp during hair relaxing.

128. _____ require the application of protective base cream to the entire scalp prior to the application of the relaxer.

129. _____ do not require application of a protective base. They contain a protective base cream that is designed to melt at body temperature.

130. List the different strengths of hydroxide relaxers and what each is formulated for.

a) _____

_____

b) _____

_____

c) _____

_____

131. Periodic _____ during processing will help inform you when the hair is sufficiently relaxed.

132. _____ is an acid-alkali neutralization that neutralizes (deactivates) the alkaline residues left in the hair by a hydroxide relaxer and lowers the pH of the hair and scalp.

133. The neutralization of hydroxide relaxers involves oxidation.

_____ True   _____ False

134. What does the application of an acid-balanced shampoo or normalizing lotion do?

_____

_____

135. In a virgin relaxer application, the application of product starts ¼ inch to ½ inch away from the scalp to the ends.

_____ True   _____ False

136. To avoid overprocessing and _____ do not apply relaxer to the hair closest to the scalp until the last few minutes of processing.

137. _____ treatments contain silicone polymers and formalin or similar ingredients, which release formaldehyde gas when heated to high temperatures.

Demonstrate the Proper Technique for Curl Re-Forming (Soft Curl Permanents)

138. What does curl re-forming accomplish?

_____

139. Soft curl permanents use _____ and oxidation neutralizers just as thio permanent waves do.

140. ⓦ **ACTIVITY**: Conduct market research in your area for chemical texture services. Call at least six different salons in the area and explain you are a student conducting market research into chemical texture services. Ask when would be a good time to either visit the salon to obtain the information or to ask the questions over the phone. It is important to be aware of their business and not interrupt the salon's workflow. If the salon agrees to the interview, ask the following questions.

a) Do you perform chemical texture services, either permanent waving or chemical relaxing in your salon?

b) If no, ask why not and record their response.

c) If yes, ask which services they perform, what they charge for those services, approximately how long each service takes, and what percentage of their business is represented by that service.

After gathering the information from the local salons, prepare a summary of your findings and state which services you feel you should become proficient in performing to achieve the highest level of success in your area.

_____

_____

_____

_____

_____

_____

_____

_____

_____

Date: _____

Rating: _____

Text Pages: 668–733

why study HAIRCOLORING?

1. How often do clients who color their hair usually visit the salon?

   _____

2. One of the most creative, challenging, and inspiring salon services is

   _____.

3. Haircoloring has the potential for being one of the most _____ areas in which a stylist can choose to work.

4. List the reasons why a cosmetologist should study and have a thorough understanding of haircoloring.

   a) _____

   _____

   _____

   b) _____

   _____

   _____

   c) _____

   _____

   _____

Understand Why People Color Their Hair

5. What are a few reasons clients color their hair?

   a) _____

   _____

b) _____

_____

c) _____

_____

d) _____

_____

e) _____

_____

Review Hair Facts

6. In addition to the desired results, what is the determining factor in choosing which haircolor to use that will affect the quality and ultimate success of the service?

_____

7. Name and describe the three main parts of the hair.

1) _____

_____

2) _____

_____

3) _____

_____

8. Which part of the hair contains the natural pigment? _____

9. The natural color of hair is determined by this substance. _____.

10. Hair _____ is determined by the diameter of an individual hair strand.

11. In fine hair, the melanin granules are grouped more _____, so the hair takes color _____ and can look darker.

12. Which hair type can take longer to process? _____

13. Hair _____ is the number of hairs per square inch, and can range from thin to thick.

14. _____ is the hair's ability to absorb moisture.

15. Match each of the following degrees of porosity with its description.

_____ 1. Low porosity   a) Cuticle is lifted; hair takes color quickly

_____ 2. Average porosity   b) Cuticle is tight; hair is resistant

_____ 3. High porosity   c) Cuticle is slightly raised; hair is normal and processes in average amount of time

16. A strand of hair that feels smooth with a cuticle that is compact, dense, and hard has a _____ porosity.

17. Hair that is extremely _____ can process more quickly and result in a deeper hair color.

Identify Natural Hair Color and Tone

18. What is the most important step in becoming a good colorist?

_____

19. The three main types of melanin in the cortex are:

1) _____

2) _____

3) _____

20. Natural hair color ranges from black to dark brown to red, and from dark blond to light blond.

_____ True   _____ False

21. _____ is the varying degrees of warmth exposed during a permanent color or lightening process. It is also known as _____.

22. _____ is the unit of measurement used to identify the lightness or darkness of a color.

23. Haircolor levels are arranged on a scale of 1 to 10, with 1 being the _____ and 10 being the _____.

24 Gray hair does not require special attention in formulating haircolor.

_____ True   _____ False

25. What is salt-and-pepper hair? _____

_____

26. A person who has hair that is 70 to 90 percent gray usually has the most pigmented hair in which part of his or her head? _____

27. The _____ is a system for understanding color relationships.

28. A _____ color is the predominant tone of a color.

29. The law of color states that when combining colors, you will always get the same result from the same combination.

_____ True _____ False

30. _____ are pure colors that cannot be achieved by combining other colors.

31. The primary colors are _____, _____, and _____.

32. What are all colors created from? _____

_____

33. Colors with a predominance of blue are _____ colors, and colors with a predominance of red and/or yellow are _____ colors.

34. _____ is the strongest of the primary colors and is the only _____ primary color.

35. Which primary color can bring depth or darkness to any color? _____

36. _____ is the medium primary color.

37. Red added to blue-based colors will cause them to appear:

_____ a) darker. _____ c) white.

_____ b) lighter. _____ d) black.

38. Red added to yellow colors will cause them to become:

_____ a) darker. _____ c) white.

_____ b) lighter. _____ d) black.

39. The weakest of the primary colors is _____.

40. When you add yellow to other colors, the resulting color will look:

_____ a) deeper and darker. _____ c) more youthful.

_____ b) lighter and brighter. _____ d) more sophisticated.

41. When all three primary colors are present in equal proportions, the resulting color is _____.

42. A _____ color is a color obtained by mixing equal parts of two primary colors.

43. The secondary colors are _____, _____, and _____.

44. Green is an equal combination of _____ and _____.

45. Orange is an equal combination of _____ and _____.

46. Violet is an equal combination of _____ and _____.

47. A _____ is an intermediate color achieved by mixing a secondary color and its neighboring primary color on the color wheel in _____ amounts.

48. Tertiary colors include:

a) _____

b) _____

c) _____

d) _____

e) _____

f) _____

49. _____ are primary and secondary colors positioned directly opposite each other on the color wheel.

50. Next to each of the following colors, list its complementary color.

Blue _____

Red _____

Yellow _____

51. Complementary colors _____ each other.

52. Place a P, S, and T on the color wheel in their proper places to signify primary, secondary, and tertiary colors.

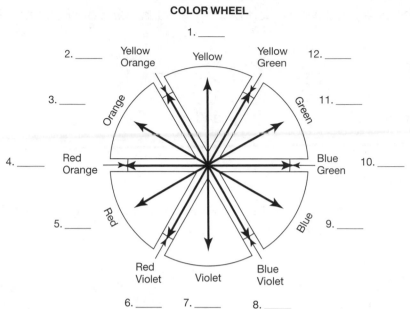

COLOR WHEEL

1. _____

2. _____ Yellow Orange   Yellow   Yellow Green   12. _____

3. _____ Orange   Green   11. _____

4. _____ Red Orange   Blue Green   10. _____

5. _____ Red   Blue   9. _____

6. _____ Red Violet   Violet   Blue Violet   8. _____

7. _____

1. _____   7. _____
2. _____   8. _____
3. _____   9. _____
4. _____   10. _____
5. _____   11. _____
6. _____   12. _____

53. What color would you use to balance hair that is orange?

_____

54. What color would you use to balance hair that is green?

_____

55. What color would you use to balance hair that is yellow?

_____

56. _____, or the hue, refers to the balance of the color and can be described as _____, _____, or _____.

57. _____ tones reflect light so they look lighter than their actual level. These tones are:

a) _____

b) _____

c) _____

d) _____

58. _____ tones are colors that absorb more light, therefore they look deeper than their actual level. These tones are:

a) _____

b) _____

c) _____

59. _____ tones are warm tones and are described as _____ or _____.

60. The strength of a color can be described as soft, medium, or strong. Color _____ are tones that can be added to a haircolor formula to intensify the result.

61. A _____ is the predominant tone of a color.

62. What base color is often used to cover gray hair?

_____

Understand the Types of Haircolor

63. What two categories do haircoloring products generally fall into?

_____

64. The oxidative category has two classifications: _____; the non-oxidative category also has two classifications: _____

_____.

65. What do all permanent haircolor products and lighteners contain?

_____

66. What are the three roles of ammonia or an ammonia substitute?

1) _____

2) _____

3) _____

67. When the haircolor containing the alkalizing ingredient is combined with the developer, the peroxide becomes alkaline and decomposes, or breaks up; lightening occurs when the alkaline peroxide breaks up or decolorizes the _____.

68. Temporary haircolors are non-oxidation colors that make only a physical change, not a chemical change, in the hair shaft.

_____ True   _____ False

69. The pigments in _____ are large and do not penetrate the cuticle layer, allowing only a coating of color is deposited which may be removed by

_____.

70. Temporary haircolor is a good choice for those who wish to _____ yellow hair or unwanted tones.

71. List the products that provide temporary hair color.

a) _____

b) _____

c) _____

d) _____

e) _____

_____

72. _____ is formulated to last through several shampoos, depending on the hair's porosity.

73. How does semipermanent haircolor work? _____

_____

_____

_____

74. The formulation for semipermanent haircolor requires mixing with a peroxide.

_____ True   _____ False

75. How long does semipermanent color usually last? _____

_____

76. Demipermanent haircolor is also known as _____ and it is formulated to _____, but not lighten color.

77. Demipermanent haircolor require both a high _____ and a high concentration of _____.

78. What is a haircolor glaze? _____

_____

79. Demipermanent haircolors are ideal for:

a) _____

b) _____

c) _____

d) _____

80. Demipermanent haircolor is available in what three forms?

1) _____

2) _____

3) _____

81. _____ can lighten and deposit color at the same time in a single process and are usually mixed with a higher-volume developer.

82. How long before a permanent haircolor service should a patch test be given?

_____ a) 12 to 24 minutes   _____ c) 12 to 24 hours

_____ b) 24 to 48 minutes   _____ d) 24 to 48 hours

83. Permanent haircolor products contain uncolored dye precursors, also called

_____.

84. Dye precursors are small and can easily _____ into the hair shaft.

85. Permanent dye molecules are trapped within the _____ of the hair and cannot be easily shampooed out.

86. What is a soap cap? _____

_____ When is it used? _____

_____

_____

87. Permanent haircoloring products are regarded as the best products for covering _____ hair.

88. Permanent haircoloring simultaneously removes _____ from the hair through lightening, while adding _____ to the hair.

89. Natural or _____ are colors obtained from the leaves or bark of plants. An example of this type of color is _____.

90. Do natural colors lighten the hair? _____

91. If a client who has used natural haircolor comes into the salon, can you apply additional chemical products over the top of natural haircolors? _____

92. _____, also called progressive haircolors, contain metal salts that change hair color gradually by progressive buildup and exposure to air, creating a dull, metallic appearance.

93. Historically, metallic haircolors have been marketed to _____.

94. What are two drawbacks of metallic haircolor? _____

_____

95. A hydrogen peroxide _____ is an oxidizing agent that, when mixed with an oxidative haircolor, supplies the necessary oxygen gas to develop color molecules and create a change in natural hair color.

96. Developers are also called _____.

97. The pH of developers is:

_____ a) between 1.0 and 2.3.   _____ c) between 6.5 and 7.5.

_____ b) between 2.5 and 4.5.   _____ d) between 8.5 and 9.5.

98. Name the most commonly used developer on the market.

_____

99. _____ measures the concentration and strength of hydrogen peroxide.

100. The lower the volume, the _____; the higher the volume, the _____.

101. Describe the common use of the following volumes of hydrogen peroxide.

a) 10-volume _____

_____

b) 20-volume _____

_____

c) 30-volume _____

_____

d) 40-volume _____

_____

102. _____ lighten hair by dispersing, dissolving, and decolorizing the natural hair pigment.

103. What happens when hydrogen peroxide is mixed into the lightener formula? _____ The process is known as _____.

104. Hair lighteners are used to:

a) _____

b) _____

c) _____

d) _____

e) _____

f) _____

g) _____

105. During the process of decolorizing, how many stages of color can the hair go through?

_____ a) 3   _____ c) 8

_____ b) 6   _____ d) 10

106. Why would a colorist choose to decolorize a client's hair before tinting?

_____

_____

107. _____ are traditional semipermanent, demipermanent, and permanent haircolor products that are used primarily on pre-lightened hair to achieve pale and delicate colors.

108. All hair will go through all 10 degrees of decolorization.

_____ True   _____ False .

109. How can you tell if you have damaged the hair during the decolorization process?

_____

_____

Conduct an Effective Haircolor Consultation

110. A haircolor _____ is the most critical part of the color service.

111. During the consultation, your client will communicate _____.
It is important that you _____ so you can make an appropriate haircolor recommendations.

112. What is the single most reliable way to ensure a client's satisfaction?

_____

113. How much extra time should you book for a client consultation?

_____

114. What is the purpose of the client intake form? _____

_____

_____

115. Wall color ideally should be _____ or _____ when performing the color consultation.

116. List some of the questions you might ask the client during the consultation.

a) _____

_____

b) _____

_____

c) _____

_____

d) _____

_____

e) _____

_____

f) _____

_____

g) _____

_____

h) _____

_____

i) _____

_____

j) _____

_____

117. How many haircolor options should you recommend to a client?

_____

118. Some medications may affect hair color.

_____ True   _____ False

119. A _____ is used by schools and many salons when providing chemical services. Its purpose is to explain to clients there is a risk involved in any chemical service and that if their hair is in questionable condition, it may not withstand the requested chemical treatment.

120. Will a release statement clear the cosmetologist of responsibility for what may happen to a client's hair? _____

Formulate Haircolor

121. List the five basic questions you should ask when formulating a haircolor.

1) _____

2) _____

3) _____

4) _____

5) _____

122. Always remember to formulate with both _____ and _____ in mind.

123. List the two methods used for the application of permanent haircolor.

1) _____

2) _____

124. When using the brush and bowl technique, the bowl should be a _____ mixing bowl.

125. When working with haircolor, you will have to determine whether your clients have any allergies or sensitivities to the mixture. To do this, you will administer a _____, also known as a _____.

126. How many hours prior to application of aniline haircolor should a patch test be given?

_____ a) 5 to 10   _____ c) 24 to 48

_____ b) 12 to 18   _____ d) 62 to 78

127. The color used for the patch test must be _____

    _____.

128. A negative skin test result will show _____.

129. A positive skin test result will show _____.

Apply Haircolor

130. How can a colorist prevent colorist dermatitis?

    _____

    _____

131. A _____ determines how the hair will react to the color
    formula and how long the formula should be left on the hair.

132. When is the strand test performed? _____

    _____

133. There is only one correct method for applying temporary haircolor.

    _____ True   _____ False

134. Semipermanent colors do not contain the _____ necessary to lift.
    So they only _____ color and do not lighten color.

135. When selecting a semipermanent color, remember that color applied on top of existing
    color always creates a _____ and alters the tone.

136. How is the application procedure for demipermanent haircolor determined?

    _____

137. Why does gray hair present a special challenge when formulating demipermanent

    haircolor? _____

    _____

    _____

138. How can you solve the challenge discussed in the previous question?

    _____

    _____

139. _____ lightens and deposits color in a single application.

140. The first time the hair is colored is referred to as a _____.

141. As the hair grows, you will need to _____ to keep it looking attractive and to avoid a two-toned effect.

142. A single-process tint that contains a non-ammonia color that adds shine and tone to the hair is a _____.

143. A visible line separating colored hair from new growth is called:

_____ a) hyperpigmentation.   _____ c) line of demarcation.

_____ b) hypopigmentation.   _____ d) line of decolorization.

144. What are some other names for hair lightening?

_____

145. If a client asks for a dramatically lighter color, what has to be done?

_____

146. _____, also known as two-step blonding, is a technique to create light-blond hair in two steps.

147. Why is a wider range of haircolor possible during a double-process high-lift coloring?

_____

_____

Show How to Use Lighteners

148. What are the three forms of lightener? _____

149. Oil and cream lighteners are _____, which can be used directly on the scalp.

150. New technology has created powder lighteners that can also be used directly _____.

151. Why are on-the-scalp lighteners popular? _____

_____

152. _____ lighteners are strong enough for high-lift blonding, but gentle enough to be used on the scalp.

153. List the features of cream lighteners.

a) _____

_____

_____

b) _____

_____

_____

c) _____

_____

_____

154. _____ are powdered persulfate salts added to haircolor to increase its lightening ability.

155. What does an activator do? _____

_____

156. Excessive heat used with hair lighteners will do what to hair?

_____

_____

157. _____ are strong, fast-acting lighteners in powdered form.

158. Why should most powdered lighteners not be used for retouch services?

_____

_____

_____

159. Name the five factors that affect processing time for lighteners.

1) _____

_____

_____

_____

2) _____

_____

_____

3) _____

_____

_____

_____

4) _____

_____

_____

5) _____

_____

_____

160. To determine the processing time, the condition of the hair after lightening, and the end results, you should perform a _____.

161. What is new growth? _____

_____

162. When performing a lightener retouch, what part of the hair should you lighten first?

_____ a) New growth   _____ b) Old growth   _____ c) Mid-shaft

163. What will occur if lighteners are overlapped during a retouch?

_____

Express How to Use Toners

164. Toners are used primarily on pre-lightened hair to achieve _____ colors.

165. What type of product is often used as a toner? _____

_____

166. The _____ pigment is the color that remains in the hair after lightening.

167. As a general rule, the paler the color you are seeking, _____

_____ .

168. Why is it not advisable to pre-lighten past the pale-yellow stage?

_____

_____

Create Special Effects Using Haircoloring Techniques

169. Special effects haircoloring refers to any technique that involves _____

_____ .

170. Coloring some of the hair strands lighter than the natural color to add a variety of lighter shades and the illusion of depth is called _____ .

171. Coloring strands of hair darker than the natural color is called _____

_____ .

172. Name the three most frequently used techniques for achieving highlights.

1) _____

2) _____

3) _____

173. The _____ of highlighting involves pulling clean, dry strands of hair through a perforated cap with a thin plastic or metal hook, and then combing to remove tangles.

174. The _____ of strands pulled through the perforated cap determines the amount of hair that will be highlighted or lowlighted.

175. The _____ of highlighting involves coloring selected strands of hair by slicing or weaving out sections, placing them on foil or plastic wrap, applying lightener or permanent color, and sealing them in the foil or plastic wrap for processing.

176. _____ involves taking a narrow, $\frac{1}{8}$-inch _____ section of hair by making a straight part at the scalp, positioning the hair over the foil, and applying lightener or color.

177. In _____ , selected strands are picked up from a narrow section of hair with a zigzag motion of the comb, and lightener or color is applied only to these strands.

178. Name four different patterns in which foil can be placed in the hair.

1) _____

2) _____

3) _____

4) _____

179. The _____ or _____ technique involves the painting of a lightener directly onto clean, styled hair.

180. To avoid affecting untreated hair when using a toner on highlighted hair, choose from the following options:

a) _____

_____

_____

b) _____

_____

_____

c) _____

_____

_____

181. _____ are prepared by combining permanent haircolor, hydrogen peroxide, and shampoo.

182. When should you use a highlighting shampoo? _____

_____

183. Do you need to perform a patch test before using a highlighting shampoo?

_____

Understand the Special Challenges in Haircolor and Corrective Solutions

184. A skilled colorist will occasionally have a problem in haircolor that can't be predicted. This may be due to _____.

185. What can cause gray hair to have a yellow cast?

a) _____

b) _____

c) _____

d) _____

186. Which of the following can be used to correct undesired yellow?

_____ a) Gold-based colors   _____ c) Violet-based colors

_____ b) Tint remover   _____ d) Orange-based colors

187. Will colors at a level 8 or lighter likely give complete gray coverage? Why, or why not?

_____

_____

188. Your client's hair is about 90 percent gray. Which color range would be most flattering to this client?

_____ a) Blond   _____ b) Red   _____ c) Black

189. What considerations should be taken into account when formulating haircolor for gray hair?

a) _____

b) _____

c) _____

190. List the tips for working with gray hair.

a) _____

b) _____

c) _____

d) _____

e) _____

f) _____

g) _____

191. _____ raises the cuticle layer of gray or resistant hair to allow for better penetration of color.

192. List the rules for effective color correction.

a) _____

b) _____

c) _____

d) _____

e) _____

f) _____

g) _____

193. What are the characteristics of damaged hair?

a) _____

b) _____

c) _____

d) _____

e) _____

f) _____

g) _____

194. When dealing with damaged hair, what should occur in conjunction to the chemical service? _____

_____

195. When dealing with damaged hair:

a) _____

_____

b) _____

_____

c) _____

_____

d) _____

_____

e) _____

_____

196. _____ are used to equalize porosity.

197. The two main types of fillers are:

1) _____

2) _____

198. _____ fillers are used to recondition damaged, overly porous hair and equalize porosity.

199. _____ equalize porosity and deposit color in one application.

200. How do you select the right color filler to fix an unwanted haircolor?

_____

_____

201. A common problem with red haircolor is _____.

202. What color should natural highlights be in a brunette?

_____

203. What is the best way to achieve pale blond results?

_____

204. What might give hair a green cast? _____

_____

205. (W) **ACTIVITY:** Consider the following haircolor challenges and enter the appropriate solutions in the table below.

Haircolor Challenge	Haircolor Solution
1. Damaged hair	
2. Unequal porosity	
3. Uneven contributing pigment on pre-lightened hair	
4. Hair will not hold a final color	

5. Drab red when a hot fiery red is desired	
6. Brown hair with orange or brassy tones	
7. Lowlights that have become too blond or all one color	
8. Dull, faded color	
9. Green cast and unwanted color	
10. 40 percent of undesired gray hair	

Know Haircoloring Safety Precautions

206. List the haircoloring safety precautions. The first and last ones are provided to help you get started.

a) Perform a patch test 24 to 48 hours prior to each application of aniline-derivative haircolor. Apply haircolor only if the patch test is negative.

b) _____

c) _____

d) _____

e) _____

f) _____

g) _____

h) _____

i) _____

j) _____

k) _____

l) _____

m) _____

n) _____

o) Always wash hands before and after servicing a client.

22 HAIR REMOVAL

See Milady Standard Cosmetology Practical Workbook.

Date: _____

Rating: _____

Text Pages: 764–809

1. Facial treatments can be very relaxing and offer many improvements to the condition and _____ of the skin.

2. Proper skin care can make oily skin look _____;
   dry skin look and feel more _____; and aging skin look _____
   _____.

why study FACIALS?

3. Why do you think it is important for you to learn the basics of skin analysis?

   _____

   _____

   _____

   _____

   _____

   _____

   _____

   _____

   _____

   _____

   _____

   _____

   _____

Conduct a Consultation and Skin Analysis

4. _____ is a very important part of the facial treatment because it determines what type of skin the client has, the condition of the skin, and what type of treatment the client's skin needs.

5. The opportunity to ask a client questions about his or her health and skin care history and to advise the client about appropriate homecare products and treatments occurs during the _____.

6. Before beginning the analysis, what must the client fill out?

   _____

7. A(n) _____ is a condition that requires avoiding certain _____
   _____ to prevent undesirable side effects.

8. Last week, your client Susan just stopped taking the drug isotretinoin for cystic acne. Today, she wants an exfoliation treatment. You should:

   _____ a) provide the service as requested since she's now off the drug.

   _____ b) tell her she does not need an exfoliation.

   _____ c) explain that she needs to wait at least six months for this service.

9. List the main contraindications to receiving a skin treatment you should look for on a client's completed client intake form. The first one is provided to help you get started.

a) Use of isotretinoin (Accutane).

b) _____

c) _____

d) _____

e) _____

f) _____

g) _____

h) _____

i) _____

j) _____

k) _____

l) _____

m) _____

n) _____

10. You may perform a facial on a client who has a fever blister, as long as you avoid the lip area.

_____ True   _____ False

11. What additional information can you obtain when the client completes the client intake form that can then be transcribed onto the service record card?

a) _____

_____

_____

b) _____

_____

_____

c) _____

_____

_____

d) _____

_____

_____

e) _____

_____

_____

f) _____

_____

_____

g) _____

_____

_____

h) _____

_____

_____

i) _____

_____

_____

12. Why should client intake forms be kept separately and secured? _____

_____

Determine Skin Type During the Skin Analysis

13. Clients with combination dry skin may have which of the following conditions?

_____ a) An orange peel texture to the skin.

_____ b) A very smooth skin surface.

_____ c) Clogged pores in the nose, chin, and center of the forehead.

_____ d) Skin that appears tight and poreless.

14. Why should you remove your rings or bracelets before performing a facial on a client?

_____

_____

15. It is possible to alter a client's skin type if you use the right product.

_____ True   _____ False

16. Skin that does not have visible pores would be considered _____;
another term for this type of skin is _____.

17. Why is acne considered a skin type? _____

_____

18. Acne is a disorder in which the hair follicles become clogged, resulting in infection of the
follicle with _____.

19. What are the two typical causes of hyperpigmentation of the skin?

1) _____

2) _____

Aging and Sun-Damaged Skin

20. Treatments that _____ and _____ improve the appearance of aging skin.

21. Home care programs for sun-damaged skin must be performed diligently and include products containing ingredients like _____, retinol, antioxidants, _____, and the daily use of a broad-spectrum sunscreen.

Categorize Skin Care Products

22. _____ are designed to clean the surface of the skin and to remove makeup.

23. List and describe the two types of cleansers.

1) _____

_____

_____

2) _____

_____

_____

24. Toners, also known as _____ or _____, are lotions that rebalance the pH and remove remnants of cleansers from the skin.

25. Toners may contain ingredients that help to:

a) _____

b) _____

26. Fresheners and astringents are usually stronger products with higher _____ content, and are used to treat _____.

27. How are toning products applied? _____

28. Some toners that contain alcohol may be sprayed on the face.

_____ True   _____ False

29. Describe what exfoliants do. _____

_____

30. What are the benefits of using exfoliants? _____

_____

_____

31. Cosmetologists may use products that remove dead surface cells from the

_____.

32. List the two basic types of exfoliants.

1) _____

2) _____

33. Mechanical exfoliants work by physically removing _____
buildup.

34. List some examples of mechanical exfoliants.

a) _____

b) _____

c) _____

d) _____

35. Some clients should not receive mechanical exfoliation or harsh mechanical
peeling. List the five conditions that would contraindicate using these services on
a client.

1) _____

_____

2) _____

_____

3) _____

_____

4) _____

_____

5) _____

_____

36. How do chemical exfoliants work? _____

_____

37. Popular exfoliating chemicals are _____.

38. Describe how these acids work. _____

_____

_____

_____

_____

39. Salon alpha hydroxy acid (AHA) exfoliants are often referred to as _____

_____.

40. Salon AHA exfoliants contain larger concentrations of AHA, usually around

_____ percent.

41. What are two precautions that must be taken before giving a client an AHA treatment?

1) _____

_____

_____

2) _____

_____

_____

42. _____ are another type of chemical exfoliant. They are known

as _____ or protein-dissolving agents.

43. How does an enzyme peel work? _____

_____

44. Usually, enzyme products are made using plant-extracted enzymes from papaya, pineapple, or beef by-products resulting in the following enzymes.

a) Papaya: _____

b) Pineapple: _____

c) Beef by-products: _____

45. What are the two basic types of keratolytic enzyme peels?

_____

46. List the seven ways proper exfoliation may benefit a client's skin.

1) _____

2) _____

3) _____

4) _____

5) _____

6) _____

7) _____

47. _____ are products that help increase the moisture content of the skin surface.

48. Moisturizers are mixtures of _____, also known as hydrators, which are ingredients that attract water and emollients.

49. What is an emollient? _____

_____

50. Moisturizers that are most often in lotion form and generally contain smaller amounts of emollient are for _____.

51. Moisturizers that are often in the form of a heavier cream and contain more emollients are needed by _____.

52. What is the most important habit to benefit the skin? _____

_____

53. A sun protection factor measures how _____ a person can be exposed to the sun without _____.

54. A(n) _____ or higher is considered to be adequate strength for daily use.

55. Night treatment products are usually more _____ products designed for use at night to treat _____.

56. _____ are concentrated products that generally contain higher concentrations of ingredients designed to penetrate the skin and treat various skin conditions.

57. Lubricants used to make the skin slippery during massage are called

_____.

58. What is the trend in treatment products for massage?

_____

59. _____ are concentrated treatment products used to cleanse, exfoliate, tighten, tone, hydrate, and nourish the skin.

60. Match each type of mask listed below with its intended use or description.

_____ 1. Clay-based masks   a) Contain oils, emollients, and humectants; used to moisturize dry skin

_____ 2. Cream masks   b) Contain paraffin and are melted at a little more than body temperature before application; harden to a candle-like consistency

_____ 3. Gel masks   c) Contain special crystals of gypsum

_____ 4. Alginate masks   d) Oil-absorbing cleansing masks that have an exfoliating and astringent effect on oily and combination skin

_____ 5. Paraffin wax masks   e) Used for sensitive or dehydrated skin

_____ 6. Modelage masks   f) Often seaweed based

_____ 7. Treatment cream   g) Generally applied underneath alginate masks

61. A thin, open-meshed fabric of loosely woven cotton is _____.

62. What is the purpose of gauze? _____

_____

63. _____ is sometimes used instead of gauze.

64. **ACTIVITY:** Conduct research into skin care products in three main categories: cleansers, toners, and moisturizers. Access the products used in your school as well as those in your home. You can also access information about other products by way of Internet research. Consider selecting products in the low, median, and high price range. Determine if there are common ingredients among each category. Identify what the benefits of each of those ingredients are. Make a list of the products and state which skin types each product would best serve and why. Draw a conclusion as to whether the more expensive products are more effective.

_____

_____

Learn the Basic Techniques of a Facial Massage

65. _____ is the manual or mechanical manipulation of the body by rubbing, gently pinching, kneading, tapping, and other movements.

66. What is the purpose of massage? _____

_____

67. Why do cosmetologists perform massage? _____

_____

68. To master massage techniques, you must have a basic knowledge of _____

_____.

69. A cosmetologist should only massage which portions of a client's body?

a) _____

b) _____

c) _____

d) _____

e) _____

f) _____

g) _____

70. Keep hands soft by using _____ and file and shape nails to avoid _____ your client's skin.

71. The impact of a massage treatment depends on:

a) _____

b) _____

c) _____

72. The direction of movement is always from the _____ of the muscle toward its _____.

73. Which portion of the muscle is the more movable attachment, meaning it is attached to another muscle or a movable bone or joint? _____

74. Which portion of the muscle is the fixed attachment, meaning it is attached to an immovable section of the skeleton? _____

75. What could result if the muscle is massaged in the wrong direction?

_____

76. List the basic massage manipulations.

a) _____

b) _____

c) _____

d) _____

e) _____

f) _____

g) _____

h) _____

i) _____

j) _____

k) _____

77. It is important to talk normally with your clients during a massage to help them feel more comfortable and relaxed.

_____ True   _____ False

78 A client who has which of the following conditions should not have a facial massage using vigorous or strong massage techniques.

_____ a) Diabetes.

_____ b) Rosacea and sensitive or redness-prone skin.

_____ c) Controlled high blood pressure.

79. Every muscle has a _____, which is a point on the skin over the muscle where pressure or stimulation will cause contraction of that muscle.

80. Identify the motor nerve points of the face on the illustration below.

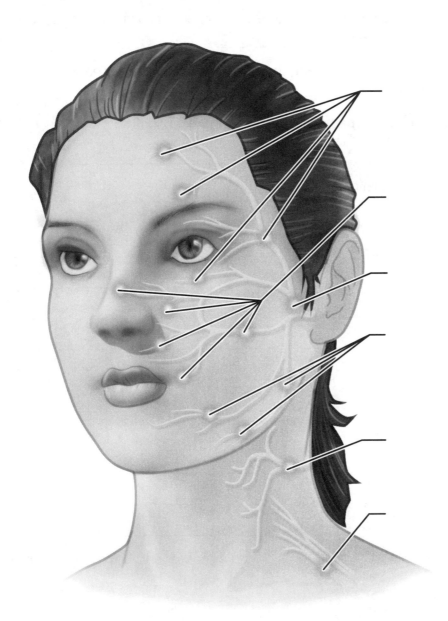

81. Identify the motor nerve points of the neck on the illustration below.

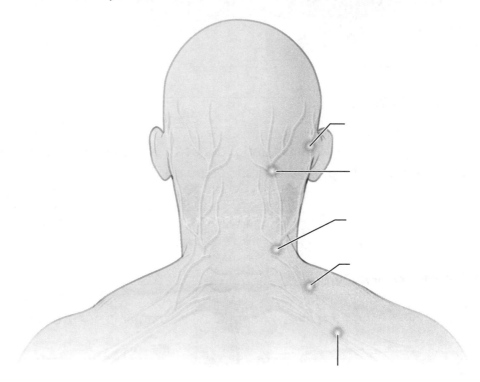

82. The following benefits may be obtained by proper facial and scalp massage:

a) _____

b) _____

c) _____

d) _____

e) _____

f) _____

g) _____

83. Once you have started facial manipulations, do not _____ your hands from the client's face until you are done with the service.

84 What is an additional consideration required when massaging a male client's face?

_____

_____

_____

Know the Purpose of the Facial Equipment

85. Facial machines will help to:

a) _____

b) _____

c) _____

86. A facial _____ heats and produces a stream of warm steam that can be focused on the client's face or other areas of the skin.

87 Steaming the skin helps to _____, making it more accepting of moisturizers and other treatment products. It also helps to _____ follicle accumulations such as comedones and clogged follicles, making them easier to extract.

88. When is steam usually administered? _____

89. What may also be used for a steam treatment if a steamer is not available?

_____

_____

90. A rotating electric appliance with interchangeable brushes that can be attached to a rotating head is a(n) _____.

91. Brushing is a form of _____ and is usually administered after or during _____.

92. What does brushing do? _____

_____

_____

93. Brushing should never be used on clients using _____

_____ or on clients who

have _____

_____.

94. The skin suction and cold spray machine is used to _____ and to jet-spray lotions and toners onto the skin.

95. Skin suction should only be used on _____ and _____ skin.

96. Spray can be used on almost any skin type.

_____ True   _____ False

How Electrotherapy and Light Therapy Treat the Skin

97. Galvanic and high-frequency treatment are types of _____, which is the use of electrical currents to treat the skin.

98. Electrotherapy should never be administered on:

   a) _____

   b) _____

   c) _____

   d) _____

   e) _____

   f) _____

   g) _____

99. An _____ is an applicator for directing the electric current from the machine to the client's skin.

100. _____ machines have one electrode and _____ have two—a positive electrode called an _____, which has a red plug and cord, and a negative electrode called a _____, which has a black plug and cord.

101. The process of softening and emulsifying hardened sebum stuck in the follicles is known as _____.

102. _____ is the process that uses galvanic current to enable water-soluble products that contain ions to penetrate the skin.

103. It is critical to always apply the passive electrode on the _____ of the client's body to avoid having the current flow through the client's heart.

104. A type of galvanic treatment using a very low level of electrical current that has many applications in skin care is _____.

105. _____ current is used to stimulate blood flow and help products penetrate the skin.

106. Electrodes for high-frequency machines are made of _____.

107. How many electrodes do high-frequency machines require?

   _____ a) 1   _____ b) 2   _____ c) 3   _____ d) 4

108. How can you prevent burns to a client during the use of galvanic current treatments?

_____

_____

_____

109. What techniques are used to apply high-frequency?

a) _____

b) _____

110. Traditionally, _____ have been used to heat the skin and increase blood flow.

111. What is a popular type of light therapy? _____

_____

112. What does an LED treatment do? _____

_____

113. What is the cosmetic use of LED light therapy? _____

_____

_____

114. A client who has a(n) _____ disorder should not receive LED treatments.

115. A type of mechanical exfoliation that uses a closed vacuum to shoot crystals onto the skin, bumping off cell buildup that is then vacuumed by suction, is known as _____.

116. Microdermabrasion is used primarily to treat surface _____ and _____.

Use Facials To Treat Basic and Specialty Skin Types

117. Facial treatments fall into two categories.

1) _____

2) _____

118. Facial treatments help to:

a) _____

b) _____

c) _____

d) _____

e) _____

119. Because skin with acne contains infectious matter, you must wear protective gloves and use disposable materials.

_____ True   _____ False

120. Home care is probably the most important factor in a successful skin care _____.

121. Approximately how much time should you block out to explain proper home care to a client? _____

122. What does a skin care program consist of? _____

_____

Use of Aromatherapy in the Basic Facial

123. Aromatherapy is the therapeutic use of plant aromas, often in the form of _____ such as:

a) _____

b) _____

c) _____

124. Many essential oils used in aromatherapy are thought to benefit and enhance a person's _____.

125. It is beyond the scope of practice for a cosmetologist to perform _____ _____ as part of aromatherapy.

126. Name three forms in which aromatherapy may be used in the salon.

1) _____

2) _____

3) _____

127. A caution when using essential oils is that too much can be _____.

Date: _____

Rating: _____

Text Pages: 810–845

1. The goal of effective makeup application is to _____ the client's individuality, rather than offering a 'make-over' based on some ideal standard.

why study FACIAL MAKEUP?

2. Explain why you think it is important to know basic makeup techniques even if you plan to focus on providing hair and chemical services to clients.

_____

_____

_____

_____

_____

_____

_____

Describe Facial Makeup and Their Uses

3. _____ is a flesh-toned cosmetic, also known as _____, that is used to minimize the appearance of skin imperfections.

4. Foundation can be used to _____

_____.

5. Foundation is available in these four forms:

1) _____   3) _____

2) _____   4) _____

6. Why would a color primer be applied to the skin?

_____

7. A client who has a yellowish or sallow skin might benefit from which color primer?

_____ a) Green   _____ c) Lavender

_____ b) Amber   _____ d) Orange

8. Most liquid and cream forms of makeup are an emulsion of _____ that act as spreading agents and help suspend various _____ _____ like titanium dioxide and iron oxides.

9. Liquid foundation is primarily _____ but often contains an emollient such as an oil or a silicone such as dimethicone.

10. Which type of finish does a foundation containing a drying agent give to the skin? _____ What does this mean?

_____

11. Foundations that are marketed as oil-free are usually intended for _____

_____.

12. _____, also known as oil-based foundation, is considerably thicker than liquid.

13. Cream foundations provide _____ coverage and are usually intended for

_____.

14. What term is most commonly used to describe a highly pigmented powder foundation?

_____

15. If a cosmetic product does not contain ingredients that would clog the follicles, it is considered to be _____.

16. All types of foundations offer some form of sun-blocking agent.

_____ True   _____ False

17. Concealers are used to hide dark eye circles, hyperpigmentation, _____ _____, and other imperfections.

18. Face powder is used to _____, making it easier to apply other powders.

19. _____ compliment eye color and are available in almost every color of the rainbow, from warm to cool, neutral to bright, and _____.

20. Eyeliner is available in pencil, liquid, _____, gel, or felt-tip pen forms and comes in a variety of colors.

21. Eyebrow pencils and _____ are used to add color and shape to the eyebrows.

22. What forms does cheek color come in?

_____

23. _____, another form of cheek color, is often added to give definition and a warm glow.

24. Lip colors are a mixture of oils, waxes, and pigments known as _____

_____.

25. What should the cosmetologist use during a facial makeup procedure to stop the lip color from bleeding? _____

26. High-performance mascaras contain _____ fibers to lengthen and thicken the hair fibers.

27. Water-based eye makeup removers are comprised of a solution to which other _____ have been added.

28. Why is greasepaint primarily used for theatrical purposes?

_____

29. A heavy-coverage pressed powder that is applied to the face with a moistened cosmetic sponge is called _____.

30. _____ is the term used for the bristles of makeup brushes.

31. The metal part of a makeup brush that holds the brush intact and supports the strength of the bristles is called a(n) _____.

32. Brush handles can be made of wood, acrylic, _____, or metal.

33. How should makeup brushes be cleaned?

_____

_____

_____

_____

_____

_____

_____

34. A smaller, more tapered version of the powder brush, is the _____
_____.

35. A lip brush is similar to the concealer brush, but with a more _____
_____.

36. A brush with firm, thin bristles that is used to apply powder to the eyebrows or eye liner at the lash line is the _____.

37. _____ may be made of velour or cotton and are used to apply and blend powder, powder foundation, or powder blush.

38. What implement is used to apply shadow and lip color or to blend eyeliner and may be used damp to intensify the eye shadow color?

_____

39. List the tips for makeup application to protect you and your client. The first one has been listed to get you started.

a) Scrape powders with clean brushes or spatulas onto a clean tissue or tray.

b) _____

_____

_____

c) _____

_____

_____

d) _____

_____

_____

e) _____

_____

_____

f) _____

_____

_____

g) _____

_____

_____

How to Use Color Theory for Makeup Application

40. The three main factors to consider when choosing makeup colors for a client are _____, _____, and _____.

41. _____ are the range of colors from yellow and gold to orange, red-orange, most reds, and even some yellow-greens.

42. _____ encompass blues, greens, violets, and blue-reds.

43. What is a neutral skin tone?

_____

_____

_____

44. Why is it not recommended to mix both warm and cool colors on the face?

_____

_____

_____

45. Neutral makeup with an orange-brown tone would be considered:

_____ a) warm neutral.   _____ b) cool neutral.

46. A complementary color for brown eyes is _____

_____.

47. A complementary color for blue eyes is _____

_____

_____.

48. The choice of color for eye makeup also depends on a person's _____

_____.

49. Why would a skin primer be applied to mature skin?

_____

_____

_____

Alter Face Shapes with Makeup

50. Face shape altering makeup creates the _____ of nearly perfect proportions wherever desired.

51. The basic rule of makeup application is that drawing light to an area _____ _____, while creating a _____ minimizes them.

52. A contour is formed when a product that is _____ than the client's skin tone is used to create shadows over prominent features so they are less noticeable.

53. The oval face is divided into three equal _____ sections. The first third is measured from the _____ to the top of the eyebrows. The second third is measured from the _____ to the tip of the nose. The last third is measured from the _____ to the bottom of the chin.

54. The oval face is approximately _____ as wide as it is long.

55. The ideal distance between the eyes is the _____ .

56. The round face is usually broader in proportion to its length than the oval face.

_____ True   _____ False

57. The _____ face is composed of comparatively straight lines with a wide forehead and square jawline.

58. A jawline that is wider than the forehead characterizes the _____ face.

59. The inverted triangle or _____ face has a wide forehead, narrow jawline, and pointed chin.

60. The diamond-shaped face has a _____ with the greatest width across the cheekbones.

61. The oblong face has greater _____ in proportion to its _____ than the square or round face.

62. For a low forehead, applying a _____ just above the brows broadens the appearance.

63. For a protruding forehead, applying a _____ over the prominent area minimizes the forehead.

64. For a _____ nose, apply a darker foundation along the _____ .

65. If the nostrils are _____, apply a darker foundation to both sides of the nostrils.

66. For a _____ nose, use a darker foundation on the sides of the nose and nostrils.

67. To balance a protruding chin and _____ nose, shadow the tip of the chin with a darker foundation and highlight the nose with a lighter foundation.

68. For a receding chin, _____ the chin by using a lighter foundation than the one used on the face.

69. For a sagging _____, use a darker foundation on the sagging portion and use a natural skin tone foundation on the face.

70. To correct a _____ jawline, highlight the thinnest areas with a lighter shade of foundation.

71. Round eyes can be _____ by extending the shadow beyond the outer corner of the eyes.

72. _____ eyes are closer together than the _____ of one eye.

73. For eyes that are too close together, create space by applying a layer of _____ _____ to the inner corners of the eyes, near the bridge of the nose.

74. Protruding or bulging eyes can be minimized by blending the _____ _____ over the prominent part of the upper lid.

75. For _____, lift the lid at the brow to reveal the natural contours. Apply a slightly deeper shadow through the crease. Blend to minimize any hard lines.

76. For wide-set eyes, apply the shadow from the _____ of the eyebrows towards the nose, and blend carefully.

77. For _____ eyes, use bright, light, reflective colors. Create a wash of color across the lid. Use a light-to-medium color along the lash line and outer corners of the eyes.

78. For _____ under eyes apply a color correcting concealer over the area to neutralize discoloration. Blend and smooth the product into the surrounding area. Set lightly with translucent powder.

79. _____ eyebrows can make the face look puffy or protruding or may give the eyes a surprised look.

80. The ideal eyebrow shape is positioned along three lines. The first line runs vertically, from the inner corner of the eye _____. This is where the eyebrow should begin. The second line runs from the _____ upward. This is where the highest part of the arch should be. The third line is drawn at _____ from the outer corner of the nose to the outer corner of the eye. This is where the eyebrow should end.

81. What should you do if the eyebrow arch is too high?

_____

_____

82. People with low foreheads should wear a _____, which would give the forehead more _____.

83. If a person has _____ eyes, build up the inside corners of the eyebrows.

84. If a person has _____ eyes, widen the distance between the eyebrows and _____.

85. If a person has a round face, arch the brows _____ to make the face appear narrower.

86. If a person has a long face, making the eyebrows almost _____ can create the illusion of a _____ face.

87. If a person has a square face, the face will appear more oval if there is a _____ arch on the ends of the eyebrows.

88. Cosmetic lash enhancers are lash lengtheners that contain _____ to make lashes look longer and fuller.

89. Lips are not positioned so that the curves or peaks of the upper lip fall directly in line with the nostrils.

_____ True   _____ False

90. What can you do for a client who has ruddy skin?

_____

_____

91. What can you do for a client who has sallow skin?

_____

_____

92. A corrective makeup technique used to conceal scars, burns, and pigmentation issues ranging from vitiligo to tattoos is called _____.

Outline the Steps for Basic Makeup Application

93. The first step in the makeup process is the _____.

94. You should _____ to the client's responses when questions are asked.

95. Describe the type of lighting that is required for a makeup consultation area.

_____

_____

_____

_____

96. Which form of artificial light is more flattering?

_____ a) Fluorescent light   _____ b) Incandescent light

97. Foundation should be as close to a client's _____ as possible.

98. If the color of the foundation is too light, how will it appear?

_____

99. If the color of the foundation is too dark, how will it appear?

_____

100. How should foundation makeup be applied to the skin?

_____

101. What is a line of demarcation? _____

_____

102. A concealer may be worn without foundation.

_____ True   _____ False

103. Apply loose powder with a large _____ or a disposable powder puff.

104. Should powder-puff applicators ever be used in the salon? Why?

_____

_____

_____

105. Why should you avoid matching an eye shadow to a client's natural eye color?

_____

_____

_____

106. Match each of the following eye shadows with its description.

_____ 1. Base color   a) Lighter than the client's skin tone and may have a matte or iridescent finish

_____ 2. Contour color   b) A medium shade close to the client's skin tone

_____ 3. Highlight color   c) Darker than the client's skin tone

107. Most clients prefer eyeliner that is the same color as the _____ or the same color as the mascara for a more natural look.

108. Lip liner color should either match the shade of the natural lip or the

_____.

109. Mascara may be used on all the lashes both at the _____.

110. When applying mascara, it is okay to double dip the wand.

_____ True   _____ False

111. When using an eyelash curler, when should you curl the lashes?

_____

Apply Artificial Eyelashes

112 _____ are eyelash hairs on a band that are applied with adhesive to the natural lash line.

113. Individual lashes are separate artificial eyelashes that are applied to the _____ one at a time.

114. List the implements and materials needed to apply false eyelashes. A few items have been provided to get you started.

    a) Adhesive tray/holder.

    b) Adjustable light.

    c) _____

    d) _____

    e) _____

    f) _____

    g) _____

    h) Hand mirror.

    i) _____

    j) _____

    k) _____

    l) _____

    m) _____

    n) _____

How to Use Special-Occasion Makeup

115. What type of makeup is most appropriate for a client who is going to be photographed with flash photography, such as at a wedding? _____

116. List the elements that should be considered when creating lips for a special occasion.

    a) _____

    _____

    b) _____

    _____

    c) _____

    _____

117. (W) **ACTIVITY:** Take some time to reflect on this chapter and think about what you learned that was significantly different than what you thought you already knew about makeup. List below five key points that you learned in this chapter that you were unaware of before. Beside each point, explain how you feel this information and knowledge will help you when you enter the field as a professional cosmetologist.

Key Point Learned	How The Information Will Aid My Career
1	
2	
3	
4	
5	

CHAPTER 25 MANICURING

See Milady Standard Cosmetology Practical Workbook.

CHAPTER 26 PEDICURING

See Milady Standard Cosmetology Practical Workbook.

CHAPTER 27 NAIL TIPS & WRAPS

See Milady Standard Cosmetology Practical Workbook.

CHAPTER 28 MONOMER LIQUID & POLYMER POWDER NAIL ENHANCEMENTS

See Milady Standard Cosmetology Practical Workbook.

CHAPTER 29 LIGHT CURED GELS

See Milady Standard Cosmetology Practical Workbook.

CHAPTER 30 PREPARING FOR LICENSURE & EMPLOYMENT

Date: _____

Rating: _____

Text Pages: 1024–1053

1. Top professionals in the cosmetology field achieved success through self-motivation, energy, and _____ _____.

2. Successful cosmetologists use their time wisely, plan for the future, go the extra mile, and draw on a reservoir of _____ to meet challenges.

why study HOW TO PREPARE FOR LICENSURE AND EMPLOYMENT?

3. List four reasons why you should study and have a thorough understanding of how to prepare for licensure and employment.

1) _____

_____

_____

2) _____

_____

_____

3) _____

_____

_____

4) _____

_____

_____

Prepare for Licensure

4. List the five factors that will affect how well you perform during the licensing examination or on tests in general.

1) _____

   _____

2) _____

   _____

3) _____

   _____

4) _____

   _____

5) _____

   _____

5. Being _____ means understanding the _____ for successfully taking tests.

6. A test-wise student begins to prepare for a test by practicing _____ and _____.

7. List effective good study habits and time management skills.

a) _____

   _____

b) _____

   _____

c) _____

   _____

d) _____

   _____

e) _____

   _____

f) _____

   _____

g) _____

_____

h) _____

_____

8. What holistic steps can you take to prepare for test taking?

a) _____

_____

b) _____

_____

c) _____

_____

d) _____

_____

e) _____

_____

f) _____

_____

9. What strategies can you adapt on test day?

a) _____

_____

_____

b) _____

_____

_____

c) _____

_____

_____

d) _____

_____

_____

e) _____

_____

_____

f) _____

_____

_____

g) _____

_____

_____

h) _____

_____

_____

i) _____

_____

_____

j) _____

_____

_____

k) _____

_____

_____

l) _____

_____

_____

_____

m) _____

_____

_____

n) _____

_____

_____

o) _____

_____

_____

p) _____

_____

_____

q) _____

_____

_____

10. _____ is the process of reaching logical conclusions by employing logical reasoning.

11. When taking a test, you should begin by eliminating options known to be incorrect.

_____ True   _____ False

12. Study the _____, which is the _____, because it will often provide a clue to the correct answer.

13. Give five examples of qualifying conditions or statements you might find in a test question.

1) _____

2) _____

3) _____

4) _____

5) _____

14. When questions include paragraphs to read and questions to answer, read the _____ first. This will help you identify the _____ information as you read the paragraph.

15. The most important strategy of test taking is to _____.

16. In true/false questions, look for qualifying words such as _____

_____; absolutes are

generally _____.

17. In a true/false statement, only part of the statement needs to be true.

_____ True   _____ False

18. Short statements are more likely to be true than longer ones.

_____ True   _____ False

19. When taking a multiple choice test, read the entire question carefully, including all the _____.

20. When answering multiple choice questions, it is wise to eliminate completely incorrect answers first.

_____ True   _____ False

21. Keep in mind that when two multiple choice answers seem similar, one of them is likely to be the _____ answer.

22. In multiple choice questions, the answer choice "All of the above" is often the correct answer.

_____ True   _____ False

23. When answering matching questions, it is best to read all items in each list before beginning.

_____ True   _____ False

24. What strategy can you use to help yourself when answering matching questions?

_____

25. When answering essay questions, make sure that what you write is _____

_____, _____, relevant to the question,

_____, and _____.

26. To be successful at test taking, you must follow the rules of _____ and

be _____ of the exam content for both the

practical and written examination.

27. To better prepare for the practical portion of the exam, you should:

a) _____

_____

_____

b) _____

_____

_____

c) _____

_____

_____

d) _____

_____

_____

e) _____

_____

_____

f) _____

_____

_____

g) _____

_____

_____

h) _____

_____

_____

i) _____

_____

_____

j) _____

_____

_____

k) _____

_____

_____

Prepare for Employment

28. Answer the following questions in your own words.

a) What do you really want out of a career in cosmetology?

_____

_____

_____

b) What particular areas within the beauty industry interest you most?

_____

_____

_____

c) What are your strongest practical skills, and in what ways do you wish to use them?

_____

_____

_____

d) What personal qualities will help you have a successful career?

_____

_____

_____

29. Your _____ is a key ingredient to your success.

30. List the key personal characteristics that will help you get and keep the position you want.

a) _____

b) _____

c) _____

d) _____

e) _____

31. "The best kind of motivation is internal." Explain why you agree or disagree with this statement.

_____

_____

_____

_____

_____

_____

32. People who take pride in their work and commit to consistently doing a good job for their clients, employers, and salon team are said to have a _____ _____.

33. Match the following type of salon with the phrase that best describes it.

_____ 1) Small independent salon

_____ 2) Independent salon chain

_____ 3) Large national salon chain

_____ 4) Franchise salon

a) Chains of five or more salons that are owned by one individual or two or more partners

b) Chain salon organization with a national name, consistent image, and business formula; owned by individuals who pay a fee to use the name

c) Salon owned by an individual or two or more partners

d) Company that operates salons throughout the country; corporate headquarters makes decisions for each salon

34. Match the following type of salon with the phrase that best describes it.

_____ 1) Basic value-priced salons

_____ 2) Mid-priced full-service salons

_____ 3) High-end image salons

a) Salons that offer higher-priced services and luxurious extras

b) Salons that depend on high volume of walk-in traffic and charge reasonable prices

c) Salons that offer a complete menu of hair, nail, and skin care services along with retail products

35. A recent cosmetology graduate is most likely to easily find a job in a(n)

_____.

36. What is possibly the least expensive way of owning one's own business?

_____

37. What guidelines should you follow when preparing your professional resume?

a) _____

_____

b) _____

_____

c) _____

_____

d) _____

_____

e) _____

_____

f) _____

_____

g) _____

_____

38. The average time that a potential employer will spend scanning your resume before deciding whether or not to grant you an interview is about _____

_____.

39. When writing a resume, you should focus on your _____

_____.

40. List the *dos* and *don'ts* of resumes. The first one has been provided to help you get started.

Dos:

a) Always put your complete contact information on your resume.

b) _____

c) _____

d) _____

e) _____

f) _____

g) _____

h) _____

i) _____

j) _____

k) _____

l) _____

m) _____

Don'ts:

a) _____

b) _____

c) _____

41. When you are marketing yourself for a job, think of yourself as a(n) _____, not just a resume.

42. A(n) _____ is a collection of photos and documents that reflects your skills, accomplishments, and abilities in your chosen career field.

43. List the elements of a powerful portfolio.

a) _____

_____

b) _____

_____

c) _____

_____

d) _____

_____

e) _____

_____

f) _____

_____

g) _____

_____

h) _____

_____

i) _____

_____

j) _____

_____

44. Once you have created your employment portfolio, it is a good idea to:

_____ a) not look at it again for a while.

_____ b) run it by a neutral party for feedback.

_____ c) mail it to all of the salons in your area.

45. 🖐 **ACTIVITY:** Using your personal computer/tablet or the school's computer lab, create a digital portfolio. Gather all the documents required for the portfolio that you learned about in this chapter and scan them into the computer. Take numerous before and after pictures of beautiful styles you have created and download them to the computer. Use your creativity to develop an appealing and effective electronic portfolio. Your work can be posted onto your personal website, personal blog, a "fan page" on your Facebook page and so forth. If you do not have access to a website, you can download the portfolio to a DVD or CD to be used when interviewing.

_____

_____

_____

46. In your own words, explain why it is a good idea to mention that you work well as a member of a team when you prepare your statement about why you chose a career in cosmetology.

_____

_____

_____

47. List the points to keep in mind when targeting potential employers.

a) _____

_____

b) _____

_____

c) _____

_____

d) _____

_____

e) _____

_____

f) _____

_____

g) _____

_____

48. A great way to find out about potential jobs is to _____ by visiting salons and talking to salon owners, managers, educators, and stylists.

49. List the guidelines to follow when networking with local salons.

a) _____

_____

_____

_____

b) _____

_____

_____

_____

c) _____

_____

_____

_____

d) _____

_____

_____

_____

50. When is it appropriate to text a salon owner or manager of a salon where you would like to work someday?

_____ a) Always; this is more effective than calling.

_____ b) Never; this is considered rude.

_____ c) Only if they request you do so.

51. If a salon rejects your request to visit, it is a negative reflection on you.

_____ True   _____ False

52. When you visit a salon, take along a _____ to ensure that you observe all the key areas that might ultimately affect your decision making.

53. After visiting a salon, remember to _____

_____.

54. Why is it important to build relationships with salons you visit, even if you decide you do not want to work there?

_____

_____

Arrange for a Job Interview

55. After targeting and observing the salon, the next step is to contact the establishments that you are most interested in by sending them a resume and requesting an interview.

_____ True   _____ False

56. You see a job you are interested in on a salon's website. How should you apply for it?

_____

_____

57. How soon after submitting your resume should you follow-up with a salon?

_____ a) The next day.   _____ b) A week later.   _____ c) A month later.

58. When preparing for an interview, make sure you have all the following items in place.

a) _____

_____

b) _____

_____

c) _____

_____

d) _____

_____

59. How many interview outfits should you have? _____

60. Your interview outfit should be _____ for the position for which you are applying.

61. Before going on an interview, make sure both your hairstyle and makeup are _____ and _____.

62. What supporting materials should you have in place?

a) _____

b) _____

c) _____

63. The following questions are typical of ones you may be asked during an interview. To prepare yourself for job interviews, answer the questions now.

_____

_____

a) Why do you want to work here? _____

_____

b) What did you like best about your training? _____

_____

_____

c) Are you punctual and regular in attendance? _____

_____

_____

d) Will your school director or instructor confirm this? _____

_____

_____

e) What skills do you feel are your strongest? _____

_____

_____

f) In what areas do you consider yourself to be less strong? _____

_____

_____

g) Are you a team player? Please explain. _____

_____

_____

h) Do you consider yourself flexible? Please explain. _____

_____

_____

i) What are your career goals? _____

_____

_____

j) What days and hours are you available for work? _____

_____

_____

k) Are there any obstacles that would prevent you from keeping your commitment to full-time employment? Please explain. _____

_____

_____

l) What assets do you believe that you would bring to this salon and this position?

_____

_____

m) What computer skills do you have? _____

_____

_____

n) How would you handle a problem client? _____

_____

_____

o) How do you feel about retailing? _____

_____

_____

p) Would you be willing to attend our company training program? _____

_____

_____

q) Would you please describe ways that you provide excellent customer service? _____

_____

_____

r) What consultation questions might you ask a client? _____

_____

_____

s) Are you prepared to train for a year before you get your own clients? _____

_____

_____

64. Some salons require applicants to _____ as part of the interview.

65. What should you bring with you to the interview if you will have to perform a service, in addition to your own model if required?

_____

66. What behaviors should you practice in connection with the interview? The first one is listed to help you get started.

a) Always be on time—better yet, be early.

b) _____

_____

c) _____

_____

d) _____

_____

e) _____

_____

f) _____

_____

g) _____

_____

h) _____

_____

i) _____

_____

j) _____

_____

k) _____

_____

l) _____

_____

m) _____

_____

n) _____

_____

67. List some questions that you might consider asking during a job interview.

a) _____

_____

b) _____

_____

c) _____

_____

d) _____

_____

e) _____

_____

f) _____

_____

g) _____

_____

h) _____

_____

i) _____

_____

j) _____

_____

k) _____

_____

l) _____

_____

m) _____

_____

n) _____

_____

o) _____

_____

68. Next to each question, indicate whether it is legal or illegal to ask in an interview:

   a) How old are you?   _____

   b) Would you describe your medical history?   _____

   c) Are you over the age of 18?   _____

   d) Are you physically able to perform this job?   _____

   e) Are you a U.S. citizen?   _____

   f) Are you authorized to work in the United States?   _____

   g) In which languages are you fluent?   _____

69. A non-compete agreement prevents you from seeking other employment
_____ after you leave employment
with your current employer.

70. A salon manager offers you a job on the spot, then hands you a non-compete
agreement. What is the best way for you to handle this?

   _____ a) Accept the job happily and sign the contract immediately.

   _____ b) Explain that you refuse to sign a non-compete agreement.

   _____ c) Ask to take it home to read it and make certain you completely understand it
            before signing it.

71. Once you are employed, take the necessary steps to learn all you can about your new
position by:

   a) _____

   b) _____

   c) _____

CHAPTER *31* ON THE JOB

Date: _____

Rating: _____

Text Pages: 1054–1075

why study WHAT IT IS LIKE ON THE JOB?

1. Working in a salon means you are a member of a(n) _____.

2. What does the term *financial management* mean to you? Why do you think it is important to understand this as a salon professional?

_____

_____

_____

_____

_____

_____

_____

_____

_____

Describe the Expectations of Moving from School to Work

3. Once you become the employee of a salon, you are expected to put the needs of _____ ahead of your own.

4. Putting the salon and the clients' needs first means:

   a) _____

   b) _____

Find the Right Position Out in the Real World

5. In a job, you will never have to do any work or perform services that are not your first choice.

_____ True _____ False

6. To be successful, you must determine which type of position is _____ by being honest with yourself as you evaluate your skills.

7. The first reality when you are in a service business is that your career revolves around _____.

8. List the five key points that will help guide you as you meet your clients' needs.

1) _____

2) _____

3) _____

4) _____

5) _____

9. Working in a salon requires that you practice and perfect your _____ and become a good _____.

10. List the workplace principles of successful team players.

a) _____

b) _____

c) _____

d) _____

e) _____

f) _____

g) _____

h) _____

11. When you take a job, you will be expected to:

a) _____

b) _____

c) _____

12. A document that outlines all the duties and responsibilities of a particular position in a salon or spa is a _____.

13. If you find yourself at a salon that does not use job descriptions, you may want to _____.

14. If you are unclear about something or need more information, it is your responsibility to _____.

15. A job description should cover:

a) _____ _____

b) _____

c) _____

16. How well you fulfill the duties listed in your job description will influence your future at the salon, as well as your _____.

17. The three standard methods of compensation in a salon are _____, _____, and _____.

18. Being paid an _____ is usually the best way for a new salon professional to start out because new professionals rarely have an established _____. Some salons offer an hourly wage that is slightly higher than the _____ to encourage new cosmetologists to take the job and stick with it.

19. If you are offered a _____ in lieu of an hourly rate, that salary must be at least equal to the _____ for the number of hours you work.

20. A _____ is a percentage of the revenue that the salon takes in from services performed by a particular cosmetologist and is usually offered once an employee has built up a loyal clientele.

21. Commissions are paid on the total _____ you generate for the salon.

22. Commissions range anywhere from 25 percent to 60 percent and are usually based on:

a) _____

b) _____

c) _____

23. A salary-plus-commission structure basically means that you receive both a _____ and a _____.

24. Another name for a salary-plus-commission is _____.

25. The salary-plus-commission structure is commonly used to _____ employees to perform more services.

26. It has become customary for salon clients to acknowledge beauty professionals with _____.

27. Tips must be tracked and reported as income.

_____ True   _____ False

28. A(n) _____ is the best way to keep tabs on your progress and to get feedback from your salon manager and key coworkers.

29. Commonly, evaluations are scheduled _____ days after hiring and then once a year after that.

30. Ask a _____ to sit in on one of your client consultations and to make note of areas where you can improve.

31. One of the best ways to improve your performance is to model your behavior after someone who is having the kind of success you wish to have, and to use that person as a _____.

32. When seeking out a role model, observe stylists who are really good and determine:

a) _____

b) _____

c) _____

d) _____

e) _____

f) _____

g) _____

33. What should you do if your mentor sees things differently than you do?

_____

_____

Manage Your Money

34. A career in the beauty industry is very _____; it is also a career that requires _____ understanding and planning.

35. The best way to meet all of your financial responsibilities is to know _____, so you can make informed decisions regarding your finances.

36. _____ is a term that means not paying back your loans.

37. One step toward making sure that you always have enough money is _____ _____.

38. Sticking to a personal _____ is a good practice to follow for the rest of your life.

39. How can you generate greater income for yourself?

a) _____

b) _____

c) _____

d) _____

e) _____

40. To get help with personal finances, you should research and interview _____ who will be able to give you advice on reducing your credit card debt, on how to invest your money, and on retirement options.

Discover the Selling You

41. The practice of recommending and selling additional services to your clients is called _____ or _____.

42. When you recommend additional salon services, you will always be the one who performs them on your client.

_____ True   _____ False

43. _____ is the act of recommending and selling products to your clients for at-home use.

44. To be successful in sales, you need:

a) _____

b) _____

c) _____

45. What is the first step in selling? _____

46. List the principles of selling.

a) _____

_____

_____

b) _____

_____

_____

c) _____

_____

_____

d) _____

_____

_____

e) _____

_____

_____

f) _____

_____

_____

g) _____

_____

_____

h) _____

_____

_____

47. A _____ involves informing clients about a product, without stressing that they purchase it. A _____ approach focuses emphatically on why clients should buy the product.

48. What are the various reasons clients are motivated to buy salon products?

   a) _____

   b) _____

   c) _____

   _____

49. Your first consideration is to always keep in mind the _____

   _____.

50. To sell a product, you will need to know exactly what your client's _____

   are, and you need to have a clear idea as to how they can be _____.

51. How can you get the conversation started on retailing products?

   a) _____

   _____

   b) _____

   _____

   c) _____

   _____

   d) _____

   _____

   e) _____

   _____

   f) _____

   _____

   g) _____

   _____

   h) _____

   _____

Keep Current Clients and Expand Your Client Base

52. Once you have mastered the basics of good service, take a look at some _____ _____ that will expand your client base.

53. List suggested marketing techniques that will keep your clients coming back to you. The first one has been provided to help get you started.

   a) Send birthday cards with reminders and promotions.

   b) _____

   c) _____

   d) _____

   e) _____

   f) _____

   g) _____

   h) _____

   i) _____

   j) _____

   k) _____

54. The best time to think about getting your client back into the salon is while they are still in your salon.

   _____ True   _____ False

55. The best way to encourage your clients to book another appointment before they leave is to _____

   _____.

On Your Way

56. Remember, your _____ job will most likely be the most _____.

57. Make the commitment to _____ your technical and customer service skills, and above all, always remain willing to _____.

58. ⚜ **ACTIVITY:** The majority of the clients you encounter will truly appreciate the work you do for them and show their appreciation for your hard work with their loyalty. In the following chart, consider the important points listed for providing excellent customer service as well as practicing workplace principles for teamwork. Rate yourself in each category on a scale of 1 to 10 with 10 meaning you are a "rock star" and 1 meaning you do not do this particular activity at all. Be honest in your evaluation and avoid selecting 5 - that's too easy. Select a rating that is either above or below 5. After rating yourself, select at least three areas that need improvement and then list three action steps you plan to take to improve it. Feel free to create an action plan for as many areas as you feel need improvement.

_____

_____

_____

Behavior	Rating	Action Planned
Put others first.		
Be true to your word.		
Be punctual.		
Be a problem solver.		
Be a lifelong learner.		
Strive to help.		
Pitch in.		
Share your knowledge.		

Remain positive.		
Become a relationship builder.	(4)	(Practice asking others questions about their interests and hobbies, and then practice active listening, allowing them to be the most important person in the conversation.)
Be willing to resolve conflicts.		
Be willing to be subordinate.		
Be sincerely loyal.		

Date: _____

Rating: _____

Text Pages: 1076–1101

1. To be successful in the beauty industry, you should be prepared to be both a great _____ _____ and a successful _ _____.

why study THE SALON BUSINESS?

2. In your own words, explain why cosmetologists should study and have a thorough understanding of the salon business.

_____

_____

_____

_____

_____

_____

_____

3. You have no future plans to own your own business. Why is it still important for you to understand the rules of business that affect salons?

_____

_____

_____

Review Types of Business Options

4. The two main options for being your own boss are:

1) _____

2) _____

5. Salon owners typically continue to work behind the chair while they manage the business.

_____ True   _____ False

6. What is a vision statement?

_____

_____

_____

_____

7. How is a mission statement different from a vision statement?

_____

_____

_____

_____

8. A set of essential benchmarks that, once achieved, help business owners realize their mission and vision are called _____.

9. What portion of the business timeline is devoted to tending to business, its clientele, and its employees?

_____ a) Year one   _____ c) Years five to ten

_____ b) Years two to five   _____ d) Years eleven to twenty

10. Why is the name you choose for your salon important?

a) _____

_____

b) _____

_____

c) _____

_____

11. List the basic factors to carefully consider when opening a salon. The first factor has been provided to help you get started.

a) Business feasibility.

b) _____

c) _____

d) _____

e) _____

f) _____

g) _____

h) _____

12. What are the elements of a good business location?

_____

13. A(n) _____ _____ is a written description of your business as you see it today and as you foresee it in the next five years.

14. A business plan is legally binding once you have signed it.

_____ True   _____ False

15. What should be included in your business plan?

a) _____

b) _____

c) _____

d) _____

e) _____

16. What is meant by *area demographics*?

_____

_____

17. You may call on the services of a(n) _____ to help you gather accurate financial information.

18. What kind of laws must be complied with when you open a salon?

_____

19. You must also know and comply with federal _____ _____ guidelines.

20. What kinds of insurance must you purchase when you open your own business?

_____

_____

21. What are salon policies?

____

____

22. **ACTIVITY:** Using the Internet and knowledge of your town or city, research viable locations for building a new salon in your community. Be sure to consider the important elements of determining a good business location: visibility, high traffic, accessibility, and parking. Once the location is found, decide on a salon name and design a business logo and business card that would be used to promote your new business. Think about what you will do to set your business apart from competitors.

____

____

____

23. What are four types of salon ownership?

1) ____

2) ____

3) ____

4) ____

24. Describe a business that is owned by a sole proprietor.

____

____

____

25. Describe a partnership.

____

____

____

26. Describe a business owned by a corporation.

____

____

____

27. What is capital?

____

28. What is a franchise?

_____

_____

_____

_____

_____

29. It is important that all franchise locations:

_____ a) are run in a similar manner.

_____ b) carry different products.

_____ c) use different logos.

30. Choosing to run a franchise will guarantee you will make a profit.

_____ True   _____ False

31. List the eight parts of a business plan.

1) _____

2) _____

3) _____

4) _____

5) _____

6) _____

7) _____

8) _____

32. If you choose to purchase an existing salon, your agreement to purchase should include the following.

a) _____

_____

b) _____

_____

c) _____

_____

d) _____

_____

e) _____

_____

f) _____

_____

g) _____

_____

h) _____

_____

i) _____

_____

j) _____

_____

33. A lease should specify the following:

a) _____

_____

b) _____

_____

c) _____

_____

34. What can you do to protect your salon against fire, theft, and lawsuits?

a) _____

_____

_____

b) _____

_____

_____

c) _____

_____

_____

d) _____

_____

_____

e) _____

_____

_____

35. To run a people-oriented business you need:

a) _____

b) _____

36. Smooth business management depends on the following factors:

a) _____

b) _____

c) _____

d) _____

e) _____

f) _____

g) _____

h) _____

37. As a business operator, you must always know where your money _____

_____.

38. Proper _____ are necessary to meet the requirements of local, state, and federal laws regarding taxes and employees.

39. _____ is usually classified as receipts from service and retail sales.

40. _____ include rent, utilities, insurance, salaries, advertising, equipment, and repairs.

41. _____ help establish the net worth of a business at the end of the year.

42. Supplies that are used in the daily business operation are _____, and those to be sold to clients are _____.

43. A good way to keep track of service records or client cards is by using a(n) _____.

Booth Rental

44. Another term for booth rental is _____.

45. In a booth rental arrangement, a professional generally:

a) _____

_____

b) _____

_____

c) _____

_____

46. Booth rental is a desirable situation for:

_____

_____

47. What are the obligations of renting a booth?

a) _____

_____

b) _____

_____

c) _____

_____

d) _____

_____

e) _____

_____

f) _____

_____

g) _____

_____

h) _____

_____

i) _____

_____

j) _____

_____

k) _____

_____

l) _____

_____

m) _____

_____

n) _____

_____

48. As a booth renter, you will not enjoy the same benefits as an employee of a salon would, such as _____.

Elements of a Successful Salon

49. How can you ensure that you will stay in business and have a prosperous salon?

   _____

50. When planning a salon's layout, maximum _____ should be the primary concern.

51. If you plan to include a spa as part of your business, the spa area should be _____ from the service area.

52. The retail area in an upscale salon should be spacious, _____ , and well lit.

53. Ideally, you should seek the advice of a(n) _____ to help you plan the layout of your salon.

54. About how long does it normally take a new salon to begin operating at full capacity?

   _____

55. The term *personnel* refers to a salon's _____ or _____ .

56. When interviewing potential employees, consider the following:

   a) _____

   b) _____

   c) _____

   d) _____

   e) _____

   f) _____

57. What are some ways you can share your success with your staff?

   a) _____

   _____

   b) _____

   _____

   c) _____

   _____

d) _____

_____

e) _____

_____

f) _____

_____

g) _____

_____

58. It is not possible to learn how to manage other people; this is a skill that must come naturally to a manager.

_____ True   _____ False

59. Name two important civil rights laws all employers must be familiar with.

1) _____

2) _____

60. The best salons employ professional _____ to handle the job of answering phones, scheduling appointments, greeting clients, and attending to the client's needs.

61. The reception area should be _____.

62. The receptionist should be _____

_____.

63. In addition to being a greeter, the receptionist handles other important functions such as:

a) _____

b) _____

c) _____

d) _____

e) _____

64. What additional tasks will a receptionist perform in the salon during slow periods?

_____

_____

65. _____ must be scheduled to make the most efficient use of everyone's time.

66. A receptionist must have the following qualities:

a) _____

b) _____

c) _____

67. The appointment book may be an actual book that sits atop the reception desk, or it may be a _____ appointment book.

68. An important part of the salon business is handled over _____ _____.

69. When using the telephone you should:

a) _____

_____

b) _____

_____

c) _____

_____

d) _____

_____

70. Incoming phone calls are the _____ of the salon.

71. It is important to answer the phone _____.

72. When booking appointments what information should you ask for?

_____

_____

73. A professional is not available at the time a client requests. How can you handle this situation?

a) _____

_____

b) _____

_____

c) _____

_____

74. When handling complaints over the phone, how should you respond?

_____

75. The tone of your voice must be _____ and _____.

Building Your Business

76. What is advertising?

_____

_____

_____

77. Advertising must _____

_____.

78. What is the best form of advertising? _____

79. List some tools you may choose to use to attract customers to the salon. The first item is listed to help you get started.

a) Newspaper ads and coupons.

b) _____

_____

c) _____

_____

d) _____

_____

e) _____

_____

f) _____

_____

g) _____

_____

h) _____

_____

i) _____

_____

j) _____

_____

k) _____

_____

_____

l) _____

_____

m) _____

_____

n) _____

_____

o) _____

_____

80. An important aspect of a salon's financial success revolves around _____ _____, cross promoting, and _____.

NOTES